PATHOPHYSIOLOGY OF NONALCOHOLIC STEATOHEPATITIS

PATHOPHYSIOLOGY OF NONALCOHOLIC STEATOHEPATITIS

METIN BASARANOGLU
AND
BRENT A. NEUSCHWANDER-TETRI

Nova Biomedical Books
New York

Copyright © 2009 by Nova Science Publishers, Inc.

All rights reserved. No part of this book may be reproduced, stored in a retrieval system or transmitted in any form or by any means: electronic, electrostatic, magnetic, tape, mechanical photocopying, recording or otherwise without the written permission of the Publisher.

For permission to use material from this book please contact us:
Telephone 631-231-7269; Fax 631-231-8175
Web Site: http://www.novapublishers.com

NOTICE TO THE READER

The Publisher has taken reasonable care in the preparation of this book, but makes no expressed or implied warranty of any kind and assumes no responsibility for any errors or omissions. No liability is assumed for incidental or consequential damages in connection with or arising out of information contained in this book. The Publisher shall not be liable for any special, consequential, or exemplary damages resulting, in whole or in part, from the readers' use of, or reliance upon, this material.

Independent verification should be sought for any data, advice or recommendations contained in this book. In addition, no responsibility is assumed by the publisher for any injury and/or damage to persons or property arising from any methods, products, instructions, ideas or otherwise contained in this publication.

This publication is designed to provide accurate and authoritative information with regard to the subject matter covered herein. It is sold with the clear understanding that the Publisher is not engaged in rendering legal or any other professional services. If legal or any other expert assistance is required, the services of a competent person should be sought. FROM A DECLARATION OF PARTICIPANTS JOINTLY ADOPTED BY A COMMITTEE OF THE AMERICAN BAR ASSOCIATION AND A COMMITTEE OF PUBLISHERS.

LIBRARY OF CONGRESS CATALOGING-IN-PUBLICATION DATA

ISBN: 978-1-60692-465-5

Available upon request

Published by Nova Science Publishers, Inc. ✈ New York

CONTENTS

Preface		vii
Chapter 1	Abbreviations	1
Chapter 2	Pathophysiology of Excessive fat Accumulation in the Liver in the Absence of Alcohol Abuse: NAFLD	3
Chapter 3	NASH: The Pathogenesis of Hepatocellular Injury in NAFLD	25
Chapter 4	Hepatic Fibrogenesis in NASH	47
Chapter 5	Pathophysiology of the Pathological Features of NASH	51
Chapter 6	Summary	59
References		61
Index		99

PREFACE

Rapid advances on molecular studies, manipulation of the mouse genome, the development of a number of animal models, and using these in studies of nonalcoholic fatty liver disease (NAFLD) have provided important insights into the pathogenesis of this relatively common disorder. One of the most crucial advances was to recognize the links among obesity, insulin resistance, inflammation and NAFLD. A growing body of literature has shown that insulin resistance and its liver-related consequence, NAFLD, could be the result of generalized inflammation. Genetic and behavioral factors contribute to increased visceral adipose tissue where increased oxidative stress and lipid peroxidation may contribute to dysregulated production of adipocytokines, fatty acids, and bioactive lipids. This chain of these events may contribute to local and peripheral insulin resistance, a central underlying pathophysiological process that may both cause and result from increased peripheral lipolysis and elevated free fatty acid concentrations in the circulation. Abnormally elevated free fatty acids taken up by organs other than adipose tissue, such as liver and skeletal muscle, contributes to steatosis of these organs (ectopic lipogenesis). Increased muscle and hepatocellular lipid content provides substrates for oxidative stress and lipid peroxidation, and also promotes insulin resistance in both liver and muscle by disturbing their downstream insulin signaling cascades. Insulin resistance further increases peripheral lipolysis in adipose tissue, further elevates circulating free fatty acids, inhibits hepatic fatty acid β-oxidation and increases de novo synthesis of both fatty acids and triglycerides in the liver. Excessively produced triglycerides in the liver are either stored as fat droplets or secreted into the plasma as very-low-density lipoproteins. If this complex mechanism of hepatic fat synthesis and secretion capacity is overwhelmed, excessive triglycerides accumulate within the hepatocytes and manifests as NAFLD.

A fatty liver is sensitive to hepatocellular injury and sustained injury can manifest as nonalcoholic steatohepatitis (NASH), NASH-associated cirrhosis, and NASH-associated hepatocellular carcinoma. Specific depletion of hepatic natural killer T cells with consequent proinflammatory cytokine polarization of liver cytokine production might be one reason for this increased hepatic sensitivity against various stimuli. Only a minority of patients with NAFLD have the necroinflammatory changes of NASH. The development of NASH in patients with NAFLD may be the consequence of secondary abnormalities such as injured and dysfunctional mitochondria, generation of reactive oxygen species with down-regulation or consumption of antioxidants causing oxidative stress and lipid peroxidation, increased activity of cytochrome P450 2E1, disturbed production of adipocytokines, and the effects of gut-derived cytotoxic products. The dynamic interplay of these processes in the pathogenesis of NAFLD remains incompletely understood and is an area of active research.

Chapter 1

ABBREVIATIONS

AdipoR, adiponectin receptor; αSMA; α-smooth muscle actin; AOX, acyl-CoA oxidase; apoB 100, apolipoprotein B100; APS, adaptor protein with a PH (pleckstrin homology) and SH2 (Src homology 2) domain; BMI, body mass index; ChREBP, carbohydrate response element binding protein; CIS, cytokine-inducible src homology 2 domain-containing protein; CPT, carnitine palmitoyltransferase; CRP, C-reactive protein; CTGF, connective tissue growth factor; CYP, cytochrome P450; DNL, de novo lipogenesis; ECM, extracellular matrix components; GLUT, glucose transporter; HCC, hepatocellular carcinoma; HSC, hepatic stellate cells; HSP, heat shock protein; JNK, c-Jun N-terminal kinase; *HFE*, hemochromatosis gene; IDL, intermediate density lipoproteins; IKK-β, inhibitor κB kinase β; IL, interleukin; iNOS, inducible nitric oxide synthase; IRS, insulin receptor substrate; LPS, lipopolysaccharide; LXR-α, liver X receptor- α; MAPK, mitogen-activated protein kinase; MCD, methionine-choline deficient; MMC, megamitochondria with true crystalline inclusions; MRC, mitochondrial respiratory chain; MTP, mitochondrial trifunctional protein; MTTP, microsomal triglyceride transfer protein; NAFLD, nonalcoholic fatty liver disease; NASH, nonalcoholic steatohepatitis; NEFA, non-esterified fatty acids; NF-κB, nuclear factor kappa B; NKT cells, natural killer T cells; NOS2, nitric oxide synthase-2; PERPP, postendoplasmic reticulum presecretory proteolysis; PI3-K, phosphatidyl inositol 3-kinase; PKB, protein kinase B; PKCδ, protein kinase C delta; PKCε, protein kinase C epsilon; PKCλ, protein kinase C lamda; PKCθ, protein kinase C theta; PKCξ, protein kinase C XI; PPAR, peroxisome proliferator-activated receptor; PUFAs, polyunsaturated fatty acids; r-metHuLeptin; recombinant methionyl human leptin; ROS, reactive oxygen species; Ser, serine; Shc, Src homology collagen; SOCS, suppressors of cytokine signaling; SREBP-1c, sterol regulatory element-binding protein-1c; STAT-3, signal transduction and activator of transcription-3; TBARSs, thiobarbituric acid-reactive substances; TNF-α, tumor necrosis factor-alpha; TGF-β, transforming growth factor-β; UCP, uncoupling protein; VLDL, very-low-density lipoprotein; WAT, white adipose tissue.

Keywords: nonalcoholic steatohepatitis, insulin resistance, fatty acids, adipocytokines, CYP2E1, oxidative stress, mitochondrial dysfunction.

Chapter 2

PATHOPHYSIOLOGY OF EXCESSIVE FAT ACCUMULATION IN THE LIVER IN THE ABSENCE OF ALCOHOL ABUSE: NAFLD

Excessive accumulation of triglycerides in hepatocytes in the absence of significant alcohol consumption, defined as > 5% fat by weight, [1,2] occurs in about 20-30% of adults [3-8]. Excessive fat in the liver, called nonalcoholic fatty liver disease or NAFLD, predisposes to the development of nonalcoholic steatohepatitis (NASH) [1,2]. NASH constitutes the subset of NAFLD that is most worrisome because it is a significant risk factor for developing cirrhosis and its complications, including hepatocellular carcinoma (HCC) (Table 1) [9-17]. Because the accumulation of excess fat in the liver is a prerequisite for the development of NASH, understanding the underlying causes of NAFLD forms the basis for rational preventive and treatment strategies of this major form of chronic liver disease. Insulin resistance and hyperinsulinemia are the most common underlying abnormalities in people with NAFLD.

OBESITY, INSULIN RESISTANCE AND HYPERINSULINEMIA AS RISK FACTORS FOR NAFLD

Overwhelming evidence now indicates that identifying NAFLD in a patient is a sensitive surrogate marker for the presence of underlying insulin resistance in most patients [18-27]. Ideally, a balance exists between energy demand and intake in the human body. Overnutrition (obesity) and starvation are the two major abnormalities of this well preserved equilibrium. Obesity, and its consequences such as insulin resistance and the metabolic syndrome (Table 2), is a growing threat to the health of people in developed nations [27-30]. While insulin receptor defects cause severe insulin resistance, most patients with insulin resistance have impaired post-receptor intracellular insulin signaling. Moreover, there is a cross-talk among insulin sensitive tissues. For example, a single genetic defect in one insulin target tissue could result in insulin resistance in other tissues [29]. Understanding the causes and consequences of these defects is the focus of intense investigation to better understand the pathophysiology of type 2 diabetes mellitus, a common consequence of decades of insulin resistance.

Table 1. Terminology of NAFLD

NAFLD: an inclusive term for liver disease characterized by predominantly macrovesicular steatosis in which hepatocytes contain vacuoles of triglyceride
Benign or simple steatosis: the generally non-progressive form of NAFLD
NASH: the progressive form of NAFLD that also includes significant necroinflammatory changes and variable degrees of fibrosis
NASH-associated subacute liver failure
NASH-associated cirrhosis: may lose the histological features of NASH
NASH-associated HCC

Table 2. The metabolic syndrome is present when three or more of five criteria are met [422]

Abdominal obesity: waist circumference > 40 inches (men) or > 35 inches (women)
Elevated fasting glucose: ≥ 100 or treatment of elevated glucose
Elevated blood pressure: systolic ≥ 130 mm Hg or diastolic ≥ 85 mm Hg or treatment of hypertension
Elevated triglycerides: ≥ 150 mg/dL or treatment of elevated triglycerides
Low HDL-cholesterol: < 40 mg/dL (men) or < 50 mg/dL (women) or treatment

Insulin binds α-subunits of its receptor which is a cell surface receptor on the major insulin sensitive cells such as skeletal muscle, adipocytes, and hepatocytes leading to autophosphorylation of the cytoplasmic domains (β-subunits) of the receptor [29-33]. The insulin receptor has intrinsic tyrosine kinase activity activated by insulin binding and the autophosphorylated receptor activates its substrates that included insulin receptor substrate (IRS) -1, IRS-2, Shc (Src homology collagen), and APS (adaptor protein with a PH [pleckstrin homology] and SH2 [Src homology 2] domain) by tyrosine phosphorylation. These phosphorylated docking proteins bind and activate several downstream components of the insulin signaling pathways. For example, tyrosine phosphorylated Shc, with Grb2-SOS, activates mitogen-activated protein kinase (MAPK) cascade. MAPK regulates gene expression and is involved in cellular growth. Activated IRS-1 associates with phosphatidyl inositol 3-kinase (PI3-K), which then activates Akt. In both skeletal muscle and adipose tissue, these insulin-mediated phosphorylation-dephosphorylation signaling cascades induce the translocation of glucose transporters (GLUT), predominantly GLUT4 - containing vesicles, from intracellular storage sites to the plasma membrane, increasing glucose uptake to prevent abnormal glucose and insulin elevations in the plasma (insulin-stimulated glucose transport). These events and insulin-dependent inhibition of hepatic glucose output maintain glucose homeostasis. Insulin also affects glucose homeostasis indirectly by its regulatory effect on lipid metabolism. Any interference in this insulin signaling pathway causes glucotoxicity, insulin resistance and, when islet beta cells are capable of responding, compensatory hyperinsulinemia.

Hepatic expression of insulin receptor protein in humans and the levels of both IRS-1 and IRS-2 in animals were decreased in chronic hyperinsulinemic states [34-36]. Interestingly, near total to total ablation of insulin receptor protein expression in the liver (up to 95%) did not alter the hepatic glucose production in mice [36] while liver-specific insulin receptor deficient mice showed both insulin resistance and glucose intolerance [37]. It was also demonstrated in mice that hepatic IRS-1 and IRS-2 play complementary roles in the regulation of hepatic metabolism. IRS-1 was more closely linked to glucose homeostasis with the regulation of glucokinase expression while IRS-2 was more closely linked to the lipogenesis with the regulation of lipogenic enzymes SREBP-1c (sterol regulatory element-binding protein-1c) and fatty acid synthase [35].

Additional physiological roles of insulin include regulating the metabolism of macronutrients and stimulating cellular growth (Figure 1). Insulin activates synthesis and inhibits catabolism of lipids while shutting off the synthesis of glucose in the liver. Adipose tissue is one of the major insulin sensitive organs in human body and the process of differentiation of preadipocytes to adipocytes, induced by insulin, is called as adipogenesis [30,31,38-42]. Within the adipose tissue, insulin stimulates triglyceride synthesis (lipogenesis) and inhibits lipolysis by upregulating lipoprotein lipase activity which is the most sensitive pathway in insulin action, facilitating free fatty acid uptake and glucose transport, inhibiting hormone sensitive lipase, and increasing gene expression of lipogenic enzymes. Insulin also induces the degradation of apolipoprotein B100 (apoB 100), a key component of very-low-density lipoprotein (VLDL), in the liver [38].

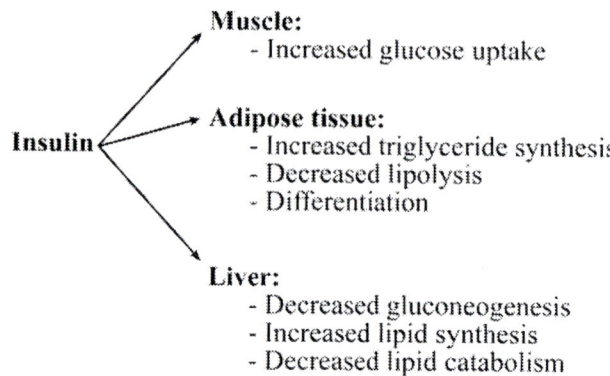

Figure 1. The major functions of insulin. Muscle, adipose tissue and the liver are the major targets of circulating insulin. Elevated insulin levels in the fed state effect a major change in whole body metabolic processes from gluconeogenesis and breakdown of fat to glucose uptake and disposal by formation of glycogen and fat while shutting off the catabolism of fat. In muscle, insulin promote glucose uptake by increasing the membrane expression of the glucose transporter GLUT4. In adipose tissue, triglyceride synthesis is increased as lipolysis and formation of free fatty acids is shut off. In the liver, gluconeogenesis and mitochondrial β-oxidation are shut off while synthesis of fatty acids and triglyceride are upregulated. These processes are impaired in the insulin resistant state such that muscle inadequately removes glucose from the circulation, adipose tissue continues to release free fatty acids even in fed state and the liver must handle this excess of fatty acids. GLUT4: glucose transporter 4.

Insulin resistance can be defined as the failure of insulin sensitive cells to respond to insulin normally. It is characterized by elevated plasma glucose and, before attrition of pancreatic β-cells develops, elevated insulin levels. Chronic hyperinsulinemia is a major contributor to glucose and lipid metabolism abnormalities. Insulin resistance diminishes the inhibitory effect of insulin on hepatic glucose output and causes impaired insulin mediated glucose uptake in both skeletal muscle and adipocytes [30,43,44]. Insulin resistance also inappropriately activates peripheral lipolysis and stimulates free fatty acid mobilization from adipocytes in the fed state. Increased circulating free fatty acids contribute to fat accumulation in the liver and muscle, further causing these tissues to be insulin resistant via disturbing their downstream insulin signaling cascades.

Cellular Mechanisms of Insulin Resistance

The most common mechanism of insulin resistance is disturbed post-receptor insulin signaling (Figure 2) [29-32,45,46]. Whereas most insulin signaling is propagated by tyrosine phosphorylation, serine (Ser) phosphorylation is often inhibitory. Ser phosphorylation of IRS-1 decreases both insulin stimulated tyrosine phosphorylation of IRS-1 (phosphorylated Ser residues of IRS-1 become poor substrates for insulin receptor) and PI3-K activation. This diminishes the downstream insulin signaling and insulin sensitivity of insulin target tissues. IRS-1 has several Ser residues such as Ser 307, Ser 612, and Ser 632 which can be phosphorylated. Prolonged insulin stimulation also causes phosphorylation of Ser residues of IRS-1 under physiological conditions [32]. Insulin and tumor necrosis factor-alpha (TNF-α) could phosphorylate the same Ser residues of IRS-1.

TNF-α and plasma free fatty acids have been shown to be major stimuli of Ser 307 phosphorylation of IRS-1 [29-32,45-49]. Inhibition of IRS-1 due to the phosphorylation of its Ser 307 residues also requires the activation of both c-Jun N-terminal kinase (JNK) and inhibitor κB kinase β (IKK-β). Both TNF-α and free fatty acids induce JNK and IKK-β activation.

TNF-α stimulates phosphorylation of Ser residues of both IRS-1 and IRS-2 in hepatocytes [46,50,51] and Ser residues of IRS-1 in muscles [47]. It was recently reported that monocyte-derived macrophages increasingly accumulated within adipose tissue of obese patients. In addition to the dysregulated production of adipocytokines by adipocytes, adipose tissue macrophages also produce proinflammatory cytokines such as TNF-α and interleukin-6 (IL-6), and C-reactive protein (CRP). Both adipose tissue and its macrophages contribute to the TNF-α burden. TNF-α functions in both an autocrine and paracrine manner. Indeed, its circulating concentrations are very low, commonly undetectable even in obese mice or humans. Thus, TNF-α may exert primarily local effects rather than distant effects [52].

Elevated free fatty acids in the circulation are also major contributors to insulin resistance in both humans and mice by stimulating Ser 307 phosphorylation of IRS-1. Adipose tissue triglycerides are the main source of circulating free fatty acids in obese. One mechanism of elevated free fatty acid-induced insulin resistance in muscle is the impaired activation of PKCλ (protein kinase C lamda) and PKCξ (protein kinase C XI) [53]. PKCδ (protein kinase C delta) and β2 might also play roles in human muscle insulin resistance. Additionally, PKCδ is reported as a possible mediator of fatty acid-induced hepatic insulin resistance [54]. In contrast, PKCε (protein kinase C epsilon), not PKCδ, is reported as a possible mediator for fatty acid-induced hepatic insulin resistance in rats (see below) [55]. Diacylglycerol, a metabolic product of long chain acyl CoAs, activates PKCθ (protein kinase C theta) which phosphorylates Ser 307 residues of IRS-1 and subsequently causes skeletal muscle insulin resistance in rodents [56]. PKCθ could also activate IKK-β which phosphorylates Ser 307 residues of IRS-1. Additionally, increased acyl CoAs or ceramide which is a derivative of acyl CoAs, promote insulin resistance by diminishing Akt1 activation [57]. Increased ceramide activates a phosphatase (protein phosphatase 2A) that reverses tyrosine phosphorylation of Akt/protein kinase B (PKB). Inactivated PKB inhibits insulin downstream signaling cascade and leading to insulin resistance in muscles [32]. It was shown in the liver of rats fed high-fat diet that activation of PKCε and JNK-1 caused the inactivation of IRS-1 and IRS-2, and eventually insulin resistance [55]. Human studies in insulin resistant patients with obesity or diabetes also pointed out a mitochondrial oxidative phosphorylation defect. Moreover, this defect was found associated with the accumulation of triglycerides in muscle [58]. Several oxidative stress mediators might also induce insulin resistance by affecting insulin downstream signaling.

Phosphatases such as PTEN, SHP 2, and PTP 1B are now recognized to be major mediators involved in insulin resistance. They dephosphorylate activated PI3-K, IRS, and the insulin receptor, respectively to induce insulin resistance. Another possible mechanism for insulin resistance is defective glucose transport such as down-regulation of GLUT4 (see above) [59].

JNK is one of the stress related kinases and plays an important role in the development of insulin resistance [46,60,61]. The three members of the JNK group of serine/threonine kinases, namely JNK-1, -2, and -3 are activated by proinflammatory cytokines such as TNF-α as well as free fatty acids and endoplasmic reticulum stress due to metabolic overload which is an intracellular abnormality found in obesity. Activated JNK induces Ser 307 phosphorylation of IRS-1, disturbs insulin downstream signaling, and subsequently causes insulin resistance. JNK activity has been found to be elevated in liver, muscle, and adipose tissue of obese experimental models [46]. Additionally, the loss of JNK-1 activity such as in JNK-1 knockout mice has been shown to prevent the development of insulin resistance in leptin deficient *ob/ob* mice or mice with high-fat induced dietary obesity.

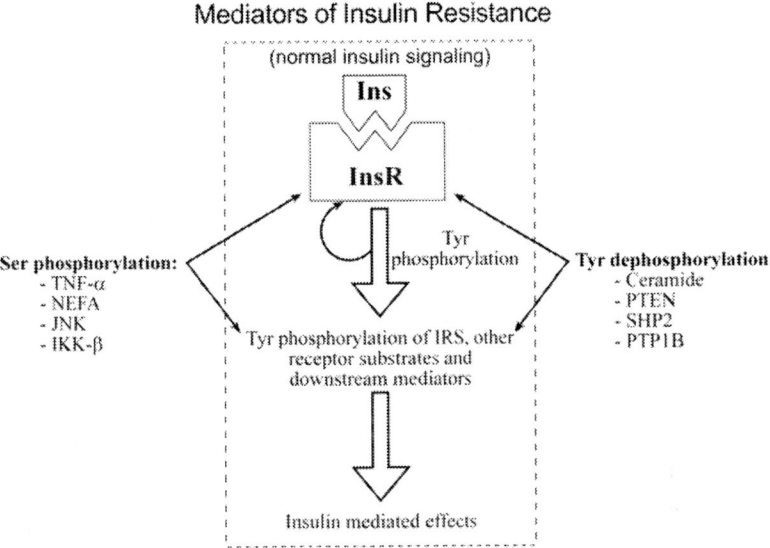

Figure 2. Major mechanisms of insulin resistance. Insulin resistance is most commonly caused by post-receptor signaling defects. The insulin receptor is a tyrosine kinase that autophosphorylates itself and also phosphorylates tyrosine residues on multiple other proteins that participate in signal transduction of the insulin binding such as the insulin receptor substrate (IRS) molecules, Shc, and APS and further downstream mediators such as PI3-K and AkT. Such tyrosine phosphorylation is required for transmitting the signal of insulin binding through the cascade of post-receptor molecules. The phosphotyrosines are dephosphorylated by a number of phosphatases, a process that is normally needed to shut off insulin signaling but can be inappropriately activated to cause insulin resistance. The receptor and the other post-receptor molecules can also be phosphorylated on serine residues, and serine phosphorylation generally impairs the functions of these proteins in transmitting the insulin signal and is a major cause of insulin resistance. Ins: insulin; InsR: insulin receptor; IRSs: insulin receptor substrates; Tyr: tyrosine; Ser: serine; TNF-α: tumor necrosis factor alpha; NEFA: non-esterified free fatty acids; JNK: c-Jun N-terminal kinase; IKK-β: inhibitor IκB kinase; PTEN: phosphatase and tensin homolog deleted on chromosome ten; SHP2: Src homology 2 containing protein tyrosine phosphatase 2; PTP1B: protein tyrosine phosphatase 1B; PI3-K: phosphatidyl inositol 3-kinase; APS: adaptor protein with a PH (pleckstrin homology) and SH2 (Src homology 2) domain; Shc: Src homology collagen.

Proinflammatory Signaling and Insulin Resistance

PKCθ and IKK-β are two proinflammatory kinases involved in insulin downstream signaling [60,61]. They are activated by lipid metabolites such as high plasma free fatty acid concentrations and there is a positive relationship between the activation of PKCθ and the concentration of intermediate fatty acid products. PKCθ activates both IKK-β and JNK, leading to increased Ser 307 phosphorylation of IRS-1 and insulin resistance. IKK-β is a mediator of insulin resistance and one of the other stress related kinases [45,62-64]. Activation or overexpression of IKK-β diminishes insulin signaling and causes insulin resistance whereas inhibition of IKK-β improves insulin sensitivity. Inhibition of IKK-β activity prevented insulin resistance due to TNF-α in cultured cells. Moreover, high-dose salicylates inhibited IKK-β activation and subsequently reversed insulin resistance in *ob/ob* mice and obese mice by a high-fat diet [45,63]. Mice heterozygous for IKK-β deletion are also partially protected against insulin resistance caused by intravenous lipid infusions, high fat diet, or genetic obesity. Evidence that this process is relevant to human disease was provided by the observation of improved insulin signaling in diabetic patients in whom high-dose aspirin inhibited IKK-β activation [65]. IKK-β phosphorylates the inhibitor of nuclear factor kappa B (NF-κB) leading to the activation of NF-κB by the translocation of NF-κB to the nucleus. NF-κB is an inducible transcription factor and promotes specific gene expression in the nucleus. For example, NF-κB regulates the production of multiple inflammatory mediators such as TNF-α and IL-6 [66]. TNF-α and reactive oxygen species (ROS) could also activate NF-κB. In contrast, antioxidants inhibit this activation. NF-κB has both apoptotic and anti-apoptotic effects. The finding that NF-κB deficient mice were protected from high-fat diet induced insulin resistance suggests that NF-κB directly participates in processes that impair insulin signaling. High-dose salicylates also inhibit NF-κB and subsequently improve insulin sensitivity. Moreover, Cai and colleagues demonstrated that lipid accumulation in the livers of obese mice due to high-fat diet led to subacute hepatic inflammation through activated NF-κB and activation of its targets, such as up-regulation of proinflammatory cytokines [66]. These subsequently promoted hepatic and systemic insulin resistance. Additionally, ROS-induced early NF-κB activation might increase the production of inflammatory mediators and cause steatohepatitis in a methionine-choline deficient (MCD) diet fed animal model [67]. The same study group also showed that these results were reversed by curcumin which inhibits NF-κB activity. Curcumin also has the ability to induce antioxidant enzymes and scavenge ROS.

SOCS (suppressors of cytokine signaling) and iNOS (inducible nitric oxide synthase) are two inflammatory mediators recently recognized to play a role in insulin signaling [68-70]. Induction of SOCS proteins (SOCS 1-7 and cytokine-inducible src homology 2 domain-containing protein [CIS]) by proinflammatory cytokines might contribute to the cytokine mediated insulin resistance in obese subjects [68-73]. In fact, the isoforms of SOCS are the members of a negative feedback loop of cytokine signaling, regulated by both phosphorylation and transcription events. SOCS-1 and particularly SOCS-3 are involved in the inhibition of insulin signaling either by interfering with IRS-1 and IRS-2 tyrosine phosphorylation or by the degradation of their substrates. SOCS-3 might also regulate central leptin action and play a role in the leptin resistance of obese human subjects [74]. SOCS might be a link between leptin and insulin resistance because insulin levels are increased in leptin resistant conditions due to the diminished insulin suppression effect of leptin because of insufficient leptin levels. Moreover, SOCS proteins might involve insulin/insulin like growth factor-1 signaling. SOCS-1 knockout mice showed low glucose concentrations and increased insulin sensitivity. In animal studies, inactivation of SOCS-3 or SOCS-1 or both in the livers of *db/db* mice partially improved insulin sensitivity and decreased hyperinsulinemia whereas overexpression of SOCS-1 and SOCS-3 in obese animals caused insulin resistance and also increased activation of SREBP-1c [70]. SREBP-1c is one of the key mediators of lipid synthesis from glucose and other precursors (de novo lipogenesis) in the liver [75]. Indeed, SOCS proteins markedly induce de novo fatty acid synthesis in the liver by both the up-regulation of SREBP-1c and persistent insulin resistance with hyperinsulinemia which stimulates SREBP-1c-mediated gene expression. These eventually cause NAFLD. Liver is the insulin clearance organ. Thus, decreased insulin clearance in patients with NAFLD further elevates insulin levels in the circulation and de novo lipogenesis rate in the liver. SOCS-1 and SOCS-3 may exert these effects by inhibiting signal transduction and activator of transcription proteins (STAT), particularly STAT-3, via binding JAK tyrosine kinase because this binding diminishes phosphorylation ability of JAK kinase to STAT-3. STAT-3 inhibits the activation of SREBP-1c. Specific STAT-3 knockout mice showed markedly increased expression of SREBP-1c and subsequently increased fat content in the liver. Conversely, inhibition of SOCS proteins, particularly SOCS-3 improved both insulin sensitivity and the activation of SREBP-1c which eventually reduced liver steatosis and hypertriglyceridemia in *db/db* mice. These results had been achieved by the improvement of STAT-3 phosphorylation and subsequently normalization of the upregulated expression of SREBP-1c [70].

Nitric oxide synthase-2 (NOS2) or iNOS production are also induced by proinflammatory cytokines [61,76,77]. High-fat diet in rats causes up-regulation of iNOS mRNA expression and increases iNOS protein activity [78]. Increased production of NOS2 might reduce insulin action in both muscle and pancreas and decreased iNOS activity protects muscles from the high-fat diet induced insulin resistance. It was also shown that leptin deficient *ob/ob* mice without iNOS were more insulin sensitive than *ob* wild-type. Thus, the production of nitric oxide may be one link between inflammation and insulin resistance. Although the concentration of iNOS was found higher in advanced stage NASH than in mild stage in obese patients with NASH [79], iNOS deficient mice developed NASH by high-fat diet [80]. The issue whether iNOS is harmful in the liver remains unestablished.

SOURCES OF LIVER FAT

Accumulation of triglycerides as fat droplets within the cytoplasm of hepatocytes is a prerequisite for subsequent events of NASH. Accumulation of excess triglyceride in hepatocytes is generally the result of increased delivery of non-esterified fatty acids (NEFAs), increased synthesis of NEFAs, or impaired intracellular catabolism of NEFAs, impaired secretion as triglyceride, or a combination of these abnormalities (Figure 3) [1]. Recent techniques such as isotope methodologies, multiple-stable-isotope approach and gas chromatography/mass spectrometry provided valuable information regarding the fate of fatty acids during both fasting and fed states [81] such as the relative contribution of three fatty acid sources to the accumulated fat in NAFLD: adipose tissue, de novo lipogenesis, and dietary (see below). Additionally, these studies reported that plasma NEFA pool is the main contributor of both hepatic-triglycerides in the fasting state and VLDL-triglycerides in both fasting and fed states (see below).

Dysregulated Peripheral Lipolysis

After a meal, insulin normally inhibits peripheral lipolysis by inhibiting hormone sensitive lipase, while reducing β-oxidation of fatty acids and increasing fatty acid synthesis from the glucose in the liver [30,44]. Moreover, under physiologic conditions, insulin inhibits the hepatic secretion of VLDL-triglycerides to the circulation by inducing apoB 100 degradation in the liver [30,82] while increased fatty acid flux into the liver increases hepatic-VLDL synthesis [83]. Additionally, free fatty acid trafficking between the adipose tissue and the liver would not cause accumulation of fatty acids in the liver under physiologic conditions. However, regulation of hormone sensitive lipase is diminished in the insulin resistant states [21,84] and lipoprotein lipase activity in adipose tissue is reduced due to the insulin resistance [30]. Hormone sensitive lipase catalyzes the hydrolytic release and mobilization of fatty acids from the increased adipose tissue triglycerides in obese subjects with insulin resistance. Increased triglyceride lipolysis enhances NEFA burden in the circulation. A recently performed NAFLD study with the combination of recent techniques (see above) showed that adipose tissue makes a major contribution to plasma NEFA pool, contributing 81.7% in fasted state and 61.7% in fed state [81]. Additionally, the contribution of dietary lipids to the plasma NEFA pool was found to be only 26.2% and 10.4% in fed and fasted states respectively in the same study. Finally, the contribution of newly made fatty acids (originating from the adipose tissue and liver) to the plasma NEFA pool was 7.0% and 9.4% for the fasted and fed states, respectively.

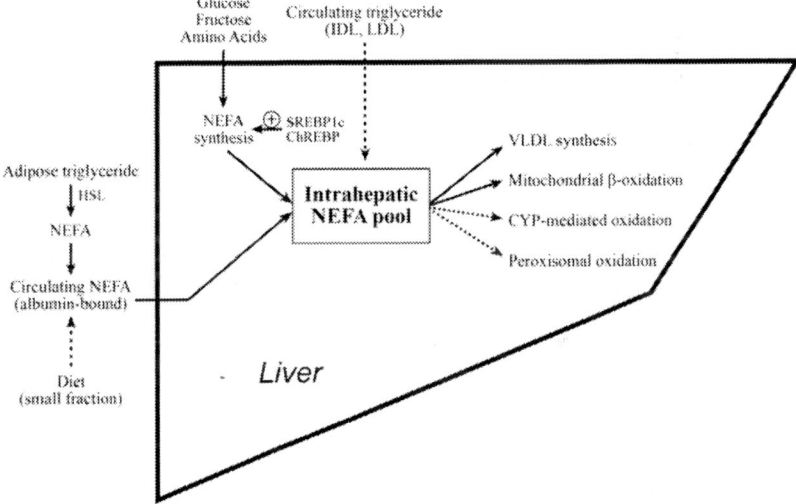

Figure 3. Sources and fates of liver fat. The major sources of fat in the liver are delivery as NEFA from adipose tissue and de novo lipogenesis from carbohydrates and amino acids. Short chain NEFA from the gut are a small fraction of total circulating NEFA in the fed state. Uptake of triglyceride in the form of LDL and IDL constitutes a minor fraction. The intrahepatic NEFA pool has two major fates. Some undergoes mitochondrial β-oxidation while most is generally re-esterified to triglyceride, incorporated into VLDL and secreted into the circulation. Catabolic pathways that contribute to the disposition of a minor fraction of NEFA include peroxisomal β-oxidation and cytochrome P450 mediated ω-oxidation. Although peroxisomal and CYP oxidation is quantitatively small, it may increase the burden of oxidant stress in the liver. NEFA: non-esterified free fatty acids; HSL: hormone sensitive lipase; IDL: intermediate density lipoproteins; LDL; low density lipoproteins; VLDL: very-low-density lipoproteins.

The liver takes up free fatty acids from the circulating NEFA pool and the rate of uptake depends only on the plasma free fatty acid concentrations. Hepatic NEFA uptake continues despite increased hepatic content of fatty acids and triglycerides [44,85] and there is no known regulatory mechanism or limitation of this process. The concentration of free fatty acids is increased in the portal circulation rapidly when the lipolysis occurs in visceral adipose tissue [30]. These products directly flux to the liver via the splanchnic circulation and contribute to hepatic triglyceride synthesis, NAFLD, and hepatic insulin resistance. Additionally, decreased adipocyte glucose uptake due to insulin resistance reduces glycerol-3-phosphate concentration in adipose tissue. This diminishes the conversion of fatty acids into intracellular triglyceride and further increases the plasma NEFA pool.

Hepatic de Novo Lipogenesis (DNL)

Hepatic de novo lipogenesis (fatty acid and triglyceride synthesis) is increased in patients with NAFLD. Stable-isotope studies showed that increased DNL in patients with NAFLD contributed to fat accumulation in the liver and the development of NAFLD [81,86]. Specifically, DNL was responsible for 26% of accumulated hepatic triglycerides [81] and 15-23% [81,86] of secreted VLDL triglycerides in patients with NAFLD compared to an estimated less than 5% DNL in healthy subjects and 10% DNL in obese people with hyperinsulinemia [87-89]. Interestingly, Donnelly and colleagues demonstrated the similarity between VLDL-triglycerides and hepatic-triglycerides regarding contributions of fatty acid sources such as 62% vs 59% for NEFA contribution, respectively; 23% vs 26% for DNL, respectively; and 15% vs 15% for dietary fatty acids, respectively in NAFLD patients [81]. These studies also showed that increased DNL in the fasting state is not increased more in fed state.

Substrates used for the synthesis of newly made fatty acids by DNL are primarily glucose, fructose, and amino acids; oleic acid (18:1, a ω-6 monounsaturated fatty acid, which is relatively resistant to peroxidation) is the major end product of de novo fatty acid synthesis. Other studies have shown that oleic acid is one of major fatty acids found in the liver in humans [90] as well as in mice with NAFLD [91]. Oleic acid is also a common dietary fatty acid type. Listenberger and colleagues demonstrated that oleic acid is readily incorporated into triglycerides and leads to the accumulation of triglycerides which was well-tolerated by cultured cells [92]. Moreover, these studies demonstrated that the cellular ability to produce triglycerides from fatty acids is strongly associated with the protection from lipotoxicity. Most importantly, this process appears a cellular adaptation mechanism against changed environmental conditions such as increased fatty acid flux into the liver in obese patients with insulin resistance. However, lipotoxicity might occur over time by chronically increased fatty acid supply when the triglyceride synthesis and storage capacity are exceeded. Palmitic acid, a saturated fatty acid, alone has no ability to incorporate into triglycerides and causes lipoapoptosis by generating both ROS and ceramides. Another crucial observation in these studies is that oleic acid generated endogenously by DNL or exogenously prevents palmitic acid-induced apoptosis. These effects had been achieved by oleic acid-inducing palmitate incorporation into triglycerides. However, lipotoxicity might occur by decreased or overwhelmed triglyceride synthesis capacity, even in oleic acid rich-medium.

Regarding NAFLD, the purpose of the increased oleic acid synthesis by DNL might be a buffer against chronically increased fatty acid supply to the hepatocytes. We might also propose that all fats in the liver might not be harmful, even they might be evidence of a protective mechanism against increased fatty acids. This might be also an explanation for whether mild degree steatosis, less than 5% fat, is important.

Although a growing body of literature suggests that NAFLD is primarily associated with a peripheral insulin resistant state, there is also a relationship between NAFLD and hepatic insulin resistance. Hepatic insulin resistance causes dysregulation of hepatic lipogenesis and fat accumulation within hepatocytes. Moreover, the contribution of hepatic insulin resistance on the development of type 2 diabetes mellitus is critical, with both increased hepatic glucose production and postprandial hyperglycemia [37,93]. One mechanism of hepatic insulin resistance in NAFLD was recently demonstrated in rats in which hepatic fat accumulation was a specific cause of hepatic insulin resistance [55]. After high-fat feeding for 3 days, rats showed increased hepatic fat content (triglycerides and fatty acyl-CoA) which originated from diet, hepatic insulin resistance, blunted insulin-stimulated IRS-1 and IRS-2 tyrosine phosphorylation, increased activation of PKCε and JNK-1, diminished insulin activation of AKT2 and inactivation of GSK3 while there was no significant peripheral insulin resistance, and no significant increase in the fat content of muscle and adipose tissue. In this model, increased hepatocellular fatty acid metabolites activated PKCε and JNK-1 which impaired IRS-1 and IRS-2 tyrosine phosphorylation and subsequently caused hepatic insulin resistance.

Elevated insulin and glucose concentrations in the plasma, abnormalities that characterize insulin resistance, independently stimulate DNL in the liver through activation of hepatic SREBP-1c and carbohydrate response element binding protein (ChREBP), respectively [94]. SREBPs are transcription factors involved in the uptake and synthesis of fatty acids [75,95-97]. The SREBP family includes SREBP-1a, 1c, and 2. SREBP-1c is predominantly located in the liver and can activate transcriptionally the genes involved in hepatic lipogenesis [75,97]. A study performed with *ob/ob* mice deficient for SREBP-1c demonstrated 50% reduction in hepatic triglyceride content [98]. Fasting reduces and feeding increases the amount of SREBP-1c in the liver. In patients with NAFLD, insulin continues to stimulate SREBP-1c mediated lipogenic genes expression despite profound insulin resistance. SREBP-1c also stimulates the expression of enzymes that produce malonyl-CoA at the mitochondrial membrane, a molecule that potently inhibits mitochondrial fatty acid uptake and β-oxidation. Fatty acids thus undergo triglyceride synthesis or oxidation in peroxisomes and smooth endoplasmic reticulum which produces more ROS. Thus, SREBP-1c activation not only favors the formation of fatty acids, but it also down-regulates their catabolism which further contributes to the formation of triglyceride.

Fatty acid synthesis is only partially (30-50%) dependent on SREBPs [99]. Another transcription factor, ChREBP, regulates the genes involved in the synthesis of fatty acids from glucose [100,101]. Elevated plasma glucose levels stimulate cytoplasmic ChREBP to enter the nucleus and bind to DNA leading to specific gene expression. For example, activated ChREBP activates liver type pyruvate kinase which increases both glycolysis to produce more citrate and stimulate DNL to produce fatty acids.

Uptake of Dietary Fat into the Liver

In the fed state, most triglyceride in the plasma is found in gut-derived chylomicrons or liver-derived VLDL. Only a small fraction of gut-derived triglyceride is taken up by the liver such that only 15% of liver triglyceride originates from dietary triglyceride while the majority originates from adipose-derived NEFA [81]. In the fasted state, triglycerides found in the plasma are primarily remnant lipoproteins such as chylomicron remnants, VLDL remnants, and intermediate density lipoproteins (IDL) [44]. Triglyceride content of remnant molecules differs between healthy and insulin resistant states because hepatic uptake is a direct function of the level of dietary fat intake, rate of hepatic secretion of VLDL, and the activity of adipose lipoprotein lipases. It was shown that high triglyceride content of remnants in insulin resistant subjects increased VLDL synthesis and secretion in both human and cultured liver cells compared to healthy controls. However, remnants were not found to stimulate VLDL secretion from the liver as much as free fatty acids.

These experimental findings are highly relevant to clinical practice. While it may be intuitive to recommend a low fat diet to patients with NAFLD, the benefit of this is primarily in reducing total caloric intake and potentially reducing cardiovascular risks. Moreover, simple sugars have the ability to stimulate lipogenesis [81,88]. Ingested carbohydrates are a major stimulus for hepatic DNL and are thus more likely to directly contribute to NAFLD than dietary fat intake. Additionally, regulation of the changes in hepatic lipogenesis from fasting state to fed state is disturbed.

Moreover, an area of ongoing research is how total caloric intake and the composition of diet affect the development of NAFLD. Studies in alcohol-fed rats showed that polyunsaturated fats are harmful and saturated fats are protective in the liver [102,103]. In contrast, a recently performed study demonstrated that not only polyunsaturated fatty acids, but also saturated fatty acids such as palmitic acid induced hepatocyte apoptosis and injury in rats [92,104]. Additionally, a low-calorie and very low-fat diet used in one study may have worsened liver inflammation [105]. This observation might be explained by the harmful effect of rapid weight loss or very low fat content of the formula [105,106]. Increased serum concentrations of free fatty acids, which could be due to obesity or rapid weight loss, were also found to be correlated with the severity of fibrosis in patients with NASH [107].

FATES OF LIVER FAT

Very-low-density Lipoprotein (VLDL) Synthesis and Secretion

VLDL is a lipoprotein complex of apoB 100, triglycerides, cholesteryl esters and phospholipids synthesized only in the liver [44,108-111]. Synthesis occurs in the endoplasmic reticulum and VLDL is exported by vesicular transport from the liver into the plasma. Lipoprotein lipases in the vascular endothelium progressively remove triglyceride from circulating VLDL to produce ILD and smaller VLDL particles. Such delipidated products can be taken up by the liver but constitute a relatively minor pathway of fat uptake in the liver. The relative contributions of fatty acids derived from adipose tissue, diet, and DNL to the triglyceride content of VLDL in fasted and fed states were 60.4% and 27.9% for adipose, respectively; 12.1% and 19.1% for diet, respectively; and 22.2% and

20.4% for DNL, respectively in patients with NAFLD [81]. The similarity between VLDL-triglycerides and hepatic-triglycerides regarding contributions of fatty acid sources was also demonstrated (see above) [81]. The plasma NEFA pool contribution derived from adipose tissue comprised the largest fraction in both fed and fasted states.

Inhibition of VLDL assembly or secretion due to any reason leads to hepatic steatosis. The factors regulating apoB 100 synthesis within the hepatocytes are not completely understood and conflicting data have been reported. ApoB 100 is synthesized and secreted proportional to the amount of available triglyceride in the liver [112,113]. Its synthesis in the endoplasmic reticulum is a rate-determining step for VLDL formation and secretion. This process is facilitated by microsomal triglyceride transfer protein (MTTP) in the lumen of endoplasmic reticulum [114]. Abnormalities of MTTP also have been found to cause hepatic retention of fats and hepatic steatosis. For example, mutations in the promoter and coding regions of the MTTP gene are associated with severe hepatic steatosis and markedly decreased plasma triglyceride levels [115].

Three pathways have been identified for the degradation of this newly synthesized apoB 100 in the liver, namely endoplasmic reticulum associated degradation of newly synthesized apoB 100, reuptake, and postendoplasmic reticulum presecretory proteolysis (PERPP) [110,111,116]. Even though apoB 100 synthesis is regulated, it is synthesized in excess and roughly 70% of newly synthesized apoB 100 is not secreted and undergoes intracellular degradation [117]. The availability of triglycerides for lipidation of apoB 100 is an important factor in preventing apoB 100 from being degraded via the proteasome [116]. PERPP degrades newly synthesized apoB 100, without any contribution of proteasome and lysosomes [116]. Both in vitro and in vivo studies demonstrated that PERPP regulates decreased apoB 100 secretion because of polyunsaturated fatty acids (PUFAs) and increased apoB 100 secretion because of saturated fatty acids [111].

Insulin promotes apoB 100 degradation and decreases hepatic VLDL-triglyceride secretion under physiologic conditions [118]. However, chronic hyperinsulinemia is associated with increased apoB 100 synthesis and increased VLDL-triglyceride concentrations in the circulation, most probably due to resistance to normal insulin action [118-122]. ApoB 100 secretion is increased (40%) in obese and NAFLD subjects, but is significantly decreased (62%) in NASH subjects compared with both obese without NAFLD (body mass index-[BMI], gender-, and age- matched subjects) and lean without NAFLD (age- and sex- matched healthy controls) subjects [109]. Correlated with these findings, the mean metabolic clearance rate of apoB 100 was significantly lower in NASH subjects when compared with both obese without NAFLD and lean without NAFLD subjects. By comparison, the mean absolute synthesis rate of fibrinogen and albumin were not decreased, even significantly increased when compared with lean subjects and similar to that of obese subjects without NAFLD, in NASH in this same study.

One mechanism of impaired VLDL secretion may be increased oxidative stress and lipid peroxidation induced by fatty acids in the liver [111]. Increased hepatic oxidative stress and lipid peroxidation stimulate PERPP to induce apoB 100 degradation and to decrease the secretion of apoB 100, and is associated with lower VLDL concentrations in the plasma [111]. Moreover, lipid peroxidation could achieve these results even in the absence of exogenous fatty acids. It was also reported that feeding rats with PUFAs, which are predisposed lipid peroxidation, led to decreased triglycerides in both the plasma and the liver while hepatic lipid peroxidation products (hepatic lipid hydroperoxides and thiobarbituric acid-reactive substances [TBARSs]) were increased and a lipid antioxidant, vitamin E, levels were decreased [123]. An antioxidant (an iron chelator or a lipid antioxidant) added to the medium decreased oxidative lipid peroxidation, improved apoB 100 concentrations, and increased VLDL-triglyceride secretion in both rat hepatoma and primary rodent hepatocytes [111]. PUFA infusion also increased hepatic lipid peroxidation and decreased hepatic VLDL secretion in mice [111]. These studies also pointed out a direct oxidative damage to apoB 100 via enzymatic or non-enzymatic pathways.

These abnormalities are correlated with the pathogenesis of NASH. Oxidative stress and -related hepatic lipid peroxidation are associated with the development of NASH in both animal models and humans. In addition to increased free fatty acid flux into the hepatocytes, increased oxidative stress and lipid peroxidation are associated with both increased degradation and decreased secretion of apoB 100 induce lipid retention and accumulation in the liver. Moreover, the finding of Charlton and colleagues of decreased apoB 100 synthesis in NASH patients (see above) [109] might be explained by the increased oxidative stress and lipid peroxidation, PERPP degradation, in patients with NASH.

Polymorphisms of the apoB100 gene may also impair VLDL secretion. Several apoB 100 gene mutations have been reported in patients with NAFLD that lead to the synthesis of truncated apoB 100 [124,125]. According to some investigators there are two types of apoB 100 deficiency related with NAFLD, namely absolute deficient type (rare) and relative deficiency (ordinary type) [108,114].

In summary, apoB 100 synthesis and secretion is increased in fatty liver subjects but this process might still not enough for a normal VLDL assembly and triglyceride secretion. This causes the accumulation of triglycerides and eventually NAFLD.

Mitochondrial β-Oxidation

Fatty acids have two major fates in the liver, namely esterification to form triglycerides that are secreted as VLDL and mitochondrial β-oxidation. Mitochondrial β-oxidation of short, medium, and long chain fatty acids involves multiple steps which include entry of long chain fatty acids into the mitochondria, a process dependent on carnitine shuttle enzymes CPT-I (carnitine palmitoyltransferase 1; an outer membrane enzyme) and CPT-II, and the β-oxidation of fatty acids to form progressively shorter acyl-CoA moieties, acetyl-CoA [126]. Then, acetyl-CoA subunits are completely degraded by the tricarboxylic acid cycle to carbon dioxide. These oxidation processes are associated with the reduction of oxidized NAD+ and FAD to NADH and $FADH_2$. Reoxidation of NADH and $FADH_2$ to NAD+ and FAD produces electrons which transfer to the mitochondrial respiratory chain (MRC) [44,126-128]. Most of the electrons of NADH and $FADH_2$ are safely transferred to oxygen to form water in a process that generates ATP through the MRC. Partially reduced oxygen molecules, termed reactive oxygen species or ROS, are constitutively generated during this process when the electrons of NADH and $FADH_2$ directly react with oxygen and may contribute to oxidant stress if endogenous protective mechanisms are overwhelmed [126].

In the fasting state of lean subjects, NEFA are released from adipose tissue, enter into the liver and are rapidly metabolized by mitochondrial β-oxidation as a source of energy. Necessary for this to occur is a state of low hepatic malonyl-CoA concentrations which is a common feature in fasting state. Malonyl-CoA is produced by acetyl-CoA carboxylase which is the first step in fatty acid synthesis. Under physiologic conditions, adipocytes of lean people store lipids after meals and release them during the fasting period [118]. In contrast, heavily lipid-laden adipocytes in obese people continue to release fatty acids in the immediate postprandial term. Consistent with the increased flux of NEFA to the liver in obese patients with NAFLD, mitochondrial β-oxidation of fatty acids in the liver is also increased and as such may contribute to increased generation of ROS and oxidant stress [126]. Although insulin and malonyl-CoA could decrease CPT-I activity in lean people, this effect might be impaired in obese people with insulin resistance.

Excessive fatty acids might use alternative pathways other than mitochondrial β-oxidation to be metabolized and cause mitochondrial injury. These include peroxisomal and cytochrome P450 (microsomal CYP) oxidation systems regulated by mainly fatty acids and insulin [44]. These alternative fatty acid oxidation systems produce more ROS and thus their utilization may be a source of oxidant stress.

Peroxisomal Fatty Acid β-Oxidation

One relatively minor fate of fatty acids in the liver is their oxidation in peroxisomes. Peroxisomal oxidation of fatty acids is the normal route of metabolism of very long chain fatty acids (fatty acids with 20 or more carbons) and dicarboxylic acids [44,129]. It might also be involved in the oxidation of fatty acids when mitochondrial β-oxidation is impaired. Peroxisomal oxidation is a four-step pathway in which electrons from the $FADH_2$ and NADH are transferred directly to oxygen. Although this increases the production of H_2O_2, peroxisomes are uniquely endowed with the enzyme catalase that eliminates this reactive oxygen molecule.

Cytochrome P450 Fatty Acid ω (Omega)-Oxidation

Lastly, fatty acids can undergo oxidation by the CYP enzymes of the smooth endoplasmic reticulum which is a relatively minor pathway for the fate of free fatty acids. CYP2E1 and CYP4A isoforms, two such enzymes, are involved in fatty acid oxidation in conditions with substrate overload such as increased free fatty acid concentrations in obesity and increased ketone bodies in type 2 diabetes mellitus. CYP4A upregulation particularly occurs in conditions with decreased CYP2E1 activity. The expression of both CYP2E1 and CYP4A mRNA and their protein levels are increased in both obese and diabetic animal models and humans [130-145]. Their hepatic activity and expression were also reported to be increased in patients with NASH due to the increased substrates, mainly fatty acids and ketone bodies, irrespective of the underlying clinical condition, diabetes or obesity [139,142,143]. The distribution of CYP2E1 is in zone 3 (perivenular) hepatocytes which is the main site of maximal hepatocyte injury in NASH [146]. Nonetheless, the capacity of this enzyme system is very low to handle fatty acids [44,146-148]. Oxidation reactions by the CYP enzymes can be major producers of ROS because of a low degree of coupling between substrate binding and their weak affinity to molecular oxygen, leading to the release of species such as superoxide anion radical, hydroxyl radicals, and hydrogen peroxide.

Peroxisome proliferator-activated receptor-α (PPAR-α), a member of nuclear receptor super family of transcription factors, regulates the genes encoding some mitochondrial and peroxisomal fatty acid β-oxidation enzymes, lipoprotein metabolism, and hepatic fatty acid transport [146,149]. Highly expressed PPAR-α is also involved in hepatocyte proliferation caused by peroxisome proliferators.

Local and Generalized Inflammation in NAFLD

In earlier studies, researchers showed that obesity is associated with low-grade chronic inflammation in both animal models and humans, and this chronic inflammation is a link between obesity and insulin resistance [61,76,150-153]. Insulin resistance is strongly associated with NAFLD. Indeed, several investigators consequently reported that obesity is strongly related with chronic macrophage accumulation within increased adipose tissue in obese mice with high-fat diet-induced or genetically-induced mice [153], and genetically-induced obese mice and human subjects [76]. Xu and colleagues also showed that inflamed macrophages are active within white adipose tissue (WAT) and this activation occurs after increased adiposity and before insulin resistance. The origin of these macrophages might be from the circulation. Macrophages can secrete TNF-α, IL-1, IL-6, and MCP-1. As mentioned previously, these cytokines promote insulin resistance in adipose tissue and eventually increase adipose tissue lipolysis which causes insulin resistance in both muscle and the liver. Weisberg and colleagues also demonstrated that adipose tissue macrophages originating from bone marrow are the major reasons of increased TNF-α expression in adipose tissue, besides significant amount of iNOS and IL-6 expression in both mice and humans [76]. These cytokines and biologically active molecules promote insulin resistance (see above) [68,154-156]. Moreover, the authors reported a positive correlation between adipocyte size and the content (%) of accumulated macrophages in adipose. Additionally, weight loss decreased adipocyte size and improved these metabolic abnormalities [76]. Lastly, Furukawa and colleagues demonstrated increased NADPH oxidase-induced oxidative stress in accumulated fat of obese mice and humans which promoted dysregulated production of adipocytokines [157]. Increased fatty acids or accumulated macrophages might be the reason of this increased ROS production within adipose tissue. These data indicate localized inflammation and systemic consequences such as insulin resistance and increased circulating free fatty acids.

Additional evidence that this chronic inflammation causes insulin resistance comes from the restoring insulin sensitivity by various anti-inflammatory agents such as high dose salicylates via IKK-β inhibiton (see above) or anti-TNF-α antibody infusion [45,63,65].

Loria and colleagues investigated non-organ-specific autoantibodies in patients with NAFLD, and reported that autoantibodies were more prevalent in patients with NAFLD than in general population [158]. Moreover, C-reactive protein levels, as an acute phase protein and inflammation marker, were reported to be elevated in patients with NAFLD and insulin resistant states [159,160]. Lastly, Albano and colleagues investigated circulating IgG antibodies against lipid peroxidation products in 167 patients with NAFLD (79 patients with simple steatosis, 74 with NASH, and 14 with NASH-associated cirrhosis) and compared with 59 age- and sex-matched control subjects [161]. The IgG antibodies were significantly higher in patients with NAFLD than in controls. Additionally, the level and frequency of these antibodies were significantly increased in subjects with advanced fibrosis or cirrhosis, but not increased in patients with steatosis alone or NASH with mild fibrosis. This recent evidence indicates that NAFLD could be the result of generalized inflammation due to oxidative stress and related lipid peroxidation.

Chapter 3

NASH: THE PATHOGENESIS OF HEPATOCELLULAR INJURY IN NAFLD

Although much is known about how fat accumulates in the liver, much remains unknown about how this causes sustained hepatocellular injury and the consequences of injury recognized as NASH and fibrosis (Figure 4). Insulin resistance and hyperinsulinemia may contribute to these pathological changes [26]. Chronically increased free fatty acid supply from the lipolytically active adipose tissue to the liver might also contribute to the development of NASH. The prevalence and the severity of NAFLD progressively increase with the number and severity of the features of the metabolic syndrome. Some have argued that the accumulation of fat in the liver is an adaptive change to insulin resistance because of correlates in animals that experience periods of prolonged fasting and intermittent feeding [162]. This argument is correlated with the findings of Listenberger and colleagues that triglyceride synthesis and their accumulation prevented fatty acid-induced lipotoxicity in cultured cells (see above, DNL, oleic acid and comments) [92].

However, the accumulation of fat within the hepatocytes sensitizes the liver to injury from a variety of causes and the regenerative capacity of a fatty liver is impaired [163,164]. These studies also showed that obese mice with fatty liver clear endotoxin less than nonobese controls [163]. This additional stressor is sometimes referred to as a "second hit" in a paradigm that identifies the accumulation of fat as the "first hit" [165]. Possible candidates for the second hit include increased oxidative stress, lipid peroxidation and release of toxic products such as malondialdehyde and 4-hydroxynonenal, decreased antioxidants, adipocytokines, transforming growth factor-β (TGF-β), Fas ligand, mitochondrial dysfunction, fatty acid oxidation by CYPs (CYP 2E1, 4A10, and 4A14), and peroxisomes, excess iron, small intestinal bacterial overgrowth, and the generation of gut-derived toxins such as lipopolysaccharide and ethanol [1,97,165]. In addition, the regenerative capacity of the fatty liver may be compromised [164,166] and an interacting network of cytokines and adipokines that regulate inflammation is disrupted [167-172].

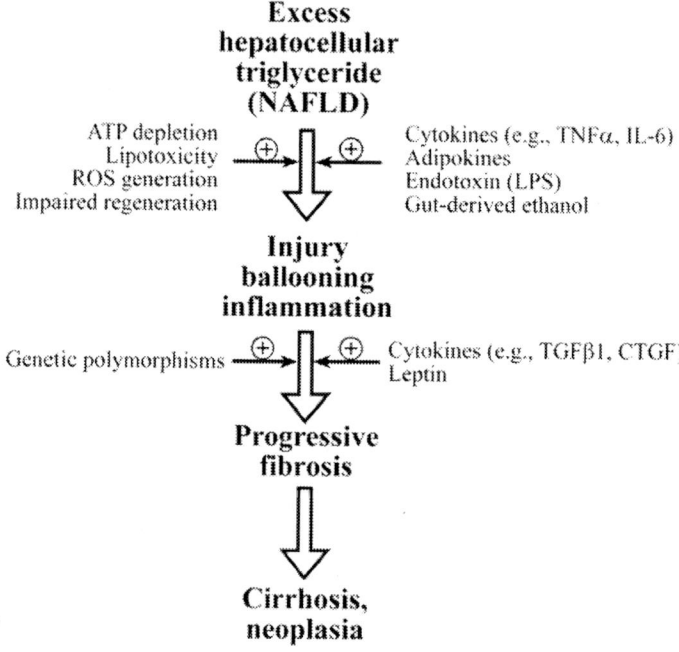

Figure 4. Possible pathway from NAFLD to NASH, cirrhosis and hepatocellular carcinoma. Multiple factors, both within hepatocytes (left side) and extracellular (right side) may contribute to injury of fat-laden hepatocytes, setting in motion the processes that lead to fibrosis, cirrhosis and hepatocellular carcinoma in some patients.

Recently, it was reported that insulin resistance is an independent predictor of advanced fibrosis in patients with NASH [26]. These findings indicate that hypoadiponectinemia, insulin resistance, and high TNF-α concentrations are not only associated with fat accumulation but also contribute to the subsequent injury found in NASH.

ROLE OF ANIMAL MODELS IN UNDERSTANDING THE PATHOGENESIS OF NASH

Understanding the molecular underpinnings of diseases accelerates the development of effective treatment and preventive strategies. Such knowledge can often only be acquired by studies of animal models that recapitulate human disease. Animal models of NAFLD and NASH have been developed and each has its strengths and weaknesses.

The ob/ob Mouse

The leptin-deficient, genetically determined, *ob/ob* mouse becomes both obese and diabetic, and develops NAFLD. This mouse strain exhibits phenotypic similarities to humans with NASH that include insulin resistance, hyperlipidemia, elevated serum TNF-α concentrations, and obesity. This model of murine liver steatosis does not progress to NASH without secondary insults such as lipopolysaccharide (LPS) treatment [173-175]. Deficiency of T-cell mediated immunity due to the lack of leptin might be the reason of these observations [176]. The *ob/ob* mouse shows up-regulated CYP4A and down-regulated CYP2E1 expression [140,177,178]. These observations are interesting because CYP4A upregulation was strongly correlated with the increased prooxidant production in a murine steatohepatitis model (CYP2E1 knockout mice fed MCD diet) (see below) [141]. Additionally, significant hepatic fibrosis may not develop in *ob/ob* mice because of the possible necessity of leptin for hepatic stellate cells (HSC) activation (see below). Furthermore, *ob/ob* mice are relatively protected from cirrhosis. Norepinephrine, a leptin-inducible neurotransmitter, activates HSC appears to be one of the major intermediate signals for this action of leptin which acts via natural killer T (NKT) cells and their products such as IL-10, a profibrogenic cytokine [174,175]. Other genetically determined obese animal models are leptin resistant diabetic (*db/db*) mice and fatty (*fa/fa*) rats.

The Methionine and Choline Deficient (MCD) Diet

One of the animal models used in many studies to further understand the pathophysiology of human NASH, particularly the source of oxidative stress mediators, is rats fed the MCD diet for 4 weeks [138] and mice fed the MCD diet for 10 weeks [141]. The MCD formula includes corn-oil which is largely unsaturated (85%). This kind of fat is an important target of oxidative stress and lipid peroxidation. Although there is a strong histological similarity between this animal model of steatohepatitis and human NASH, MCD diet fed mice are not obese and do not show insulin resistance. On the contrary, MCD diet fed mice have increased insulin hypersensitivity and their serum insulin and glucose levels are lower than wild-type mice fed standard diets (chow fed) [179]. Moreover, these mice lost weight during the experiment despite a relatively higher food intake. However, this kind of nutritional deficiency (MCD) is not common in humans.

MCD diet fed mice have increased total hepatic triglyceride content, steatohepatitis, increased hepatocyte proliferation, decreased circulating triglycerides, elevated liver enzyme levels, overexpression of hepatic CYP2E1 with no significant change in CYP4A isoforms, and increased lipid peroxides which is determined by the measurement of accumulated TBARSs in the liver (about 100-fold increase) [141,180]. Microsomal NADPH-dependent lipid oxidases may also be involved in lipid peroxidation. Mechanisms of injury that might include elevated hepatocellular lipid content which provides a large amount of substrate for lipid peroxidation, inhibition of fatty acid oxidation, induction of CYPs and induction of hepatic lipid peroxidation, could be involved in the development of steatohepatitis of MCD diet fed mice model. The role of TNF-α remains unclear in this murine model of steatohepatitis. There is also no sex hormone associated-effects [180]. PPAR-α deficiency, which causes both mitochondrial and peroxisomal fatty acid β-oxidation defects [180,181], significantly aggravated pathologic features in the liver (steatosis and steatohepatitis) in MCD diet-fed mice model [180].

Other Dietary Models

Other animal models of steatosis with or without inflammation and fibrosis have been developed by feeding mice a diet with high fat or sucrose or both with or without high caloric intake [144,145,173]. However, the type and the amount of fat of these diets have been highly variable, making comparisons difficult. Moreover, variable amounts of daily caloric intake were allowed by the investigators. A recently described rat model of feeding high-fat liquid diet (71% of energy from fat which included corn, olive, and safflower oil) for 3 weeks was reported as resemble human NASH [144]. These Sprague-Dawley rats exhibited many of the features of human NASH that included obesity, insulin resistance, hyperinsulinemia, increased hepatic TNF-α mRNA expression, induced CYP2E1 and increased CYP2E1 mRNA expression, morphologically abnormal mitochondria, increased both oxidative stress and lipid peroxidation, fatty liver, patchy inflammation, and increased collagen in the liver.

Deng and colleagues recently reported a new murine steatohepatitis model by intragastric overfeeding of male C57BL/6 mice with high-fat liquid diet for 9 weeks [145]. This formula included 37% calories from fat (corn-oil). Of the 13 mice examined, 46% had NASH features. This model showed obesity, increased WAT, insulin resistance, increased serum glucose and leptin concentrations, increased transcription of hepatic lipogenic enzymes such as PPAR-γ, LXR-α (liver X receptor- α) and SREBP-1c, decreased expression of hepatic PPAR-α, induced hepatic CYP4A with down-regulated CYP2E1, increased cytochrome reductase activity, increased hepatic mRNA expressions of TNF-α, IL-1β, IL-6, and MIP-2. These studies also reported, in WAT, increased inflammation, increased expression of both TNF-α and leptin mRNA, and decreased expression of adiponectin mRNA.

Transition from Simple Steatosis and NASH to NASH-Associated HCC: A new Murine NASH-Associated Hepatic Neoplasia Model

Xu and colleagues, recently developed a murine NASH-associated hepatic neoplasia model with the somatic inactivation of the Nrf1 gene in the livers of adult mice [182]. The authors reported that liver specific Nrf1 gene deficient mice showed similar sequence of events and the progression to histological features of human NASH. Decreased expression of antioxidant response elements containing genes and upregulation of CYP4A genes were also demonstrated. This murine hepatic neoplasia model had evidence of increased oxidative stress with the proliferation of endoplasmic reticulum before the development of liver cancer. Sustained oxidative injury and its consequences with activated hepatocyte proliferation may increase the possibility of liver cancer development in these mutant livers. This and similar models may play an important role in the further understanding of the pathophysiology of NASH and its consequences.

OXIDATIVE STRESS AND THE PATHOGENESIS OF NASH

A logical and attractive hypothesis is that oxidative stress in triglyceride-loaded hepatocytes is the cause of sustained injury with consequent NASH, fibrosis and cirrhosis [1,165,183]. The imbalance between the increased ROS and decreased antioxidants leads to lipid peroxidation of PUFAs, cellular membranes, mitochondrial membranes, and DNA [21,146,184-187]. ROS have relatively short-lived and local effects while lipid peroxidation products have longer half-lives and the capability to reach extracellular targets. Lipid peroxidation produces cytotoxic aldehydes such as malondialdehyde and 4-hydroxynonenal. ROS and these aldehydes further contribute to oxidative stress, decreased ATP production, and increased proinflammatory cytokine release. These events promote hepatocyte injury, necroinflammation, hepatocytes apoptosis, and fibrosis. Hepatocyte ballooning and the development of megamitochondria with true crystalline inclusions (MMC) might be the result of this oxidative stress and lipid peroxidation as well.

Despite the attractiveness of this hypothesis, supporting data has been sparse. Some studies have suggested a benefit of the antioxidant vitamin E [188-190], but effective antioxidants have not been rigorously tested in clinical trials. Most clinical studies only provide correlations between the presence of NASH and elevated indices of oxidant stress without establishing a causal relationship [21,146,184,187,191]. Additionally, the lipid peroxidation product 4-hydroxynonenal was found more in perivenular zone (zone 3) than periportal zone in patients with NASH, correlating with the histological lesions of NASH that are predominantly in zone 3 [187]. Moreover, more evidence of lipid peroxidation and oxidative DNA damage has been found in NASH than in simple steatosis. Lipid peroxidation was greater in patients with NASH than in patients with simple steatosis. The same study also showed that increased 4-hydroxynonenal strongly correlated with both the grade of necroinflammation and the stage of NASH, but not with the grade of steatosis while increased evidence of oxidant damage to DNA as measured by 8-hydroxydeoxyguanosine only correlated with the grade of necroinflammation in patients with NASH. This being said, oxidant stress could play a central role in causing NASH and our clinically available antioxidants may simply be ineffective at preventing the disease to prove the point. A number of sources of increased ROS production have been established in NASH that include proinflammatory cytokines such as TNF-α, iron overload, overburdened and dysfunctional mitochondria, CYPs, and peroxisomes.

Mitochondria as a Source of Oxidant Stress

The hepatocyte mitochondria are the main site of β-oxidation of free fatty acids. The electrons removed from free fatty acids during β-oxidation are shuttled through the mitochondrial electron transport chain (MRC), eventually leading to ATP synthesis and the generation of carbon dioxide and water (see above). Inherent in this process is the dissociation of partially reduced molecular oxygen in the form of superoxide, hydrogen peroxide and the hydroxyl radical, species collectively termed reactive oxygen species, or ROS. About 1%-5% of oxygen consumed during cellular respiration is not fully reduced to water during this process under physiologic conditions [192] and the production of these ROS is further increased in dysfunctional mitochondria. Thus, mitochondria have been proposed to play a central role in the pathogenesis of NASH [126].

Mitochondria also increase their oxidation capacity for the increased fatty acid flux as observed in obesity and insulin resistant states in humans and in animals fed high-fat diet. However, this increase has its limits and excess free fatty acids are metabolized at other sites in hepatocytes such as peroxisomes (β-oxidation) and the smooth endoplasmic reticulum (ω-oxidation). Acyl-CoA oxidase (AOX) catalyzes the initial reaction of fatty acid oxidation in peroxisomes, a process that generates hydrogen peroxide and thus may contribute to oxidant stress.

P450 as a Source of Oxidant Stress

Fatty acids not oxidized by mitochondria are mainly oxidized by CYP2E1, a process that further increases ROS production within the hepatocytes [146,193,194]. Other CYP isoforms that may generate oxidant stress include CYP4A family such as CYP4A10 and CYP4A14, which is less active than CYP2E1 and mainly active in the setting of low concentration or deficiency of CYP2E1 [141]. The major function of this enzyme system is to metabolize endogenous lipophilic substrates such as steroid hormones, lipophilic xenobiotics, drugs and other environmental toxins. Moreover, CYPs could metabolize and activate carcinogens. Increased endogenous substrate burden such as increased levels of free fatty acids (e.g., due to increased peripheral lipolysis in obesity) and ketone bodies (increased in diabetes) induce CYP2E1 expression in humans [139,142,143,195,196].

In normal conditions, CYP2E1 oxidation produces oxygen radicals, but the balance between these ROS and the abundance of endogenous antioxidants determines the extent of resulting oxidant stress. Initial studies demonstrated increased CYP2E1 expression in diabetic or obese rats fed a high-fat diet [132,133,136,144,145,197,198] as well as in rats and mice fed a MCD diet [138,141]. Later evidence demonstrated increased hepatic CYP2E1 expression by immunostaining of paraffin-embedded liver biopsy sections in patients with NASH [139]. In contrast, hepatic content of CYP3A was decreased in all liver sections from patients with NASH. The same study additionally showed that zone 3 steatosis, which is the typical acinar localization in NAFLD, was closely associated with increased CYP2E1 expression and in some cases extending into zones 2 and 1. CYP2E1 activity was also found to be significantly higher in nondiabetic patients with NASH than healthy controls matched for sex, BMI, and age [142]. The authors assessed the hepatic CYP2E1 activity with oral clearance of chlorzoxazone, a potent skeletal muscle relaxant and in vivo CYP2E1 probe, in this study. Only nocturnal hypoxemia and β-OH butyrate were the independent predictors of increased hepatic CYP2E1 activity. In the same study, a significant increase in the lymphocyte CYP2E1 mRNA expression was demonstrated in the NASH cohort while there was no significant correlation between increased lymphocyte CYP2E1 mRNA expression and hepatic CYP2E1 activity [196]. Increased fasting insulin and insulin resistance were shown in a nondiabetic NASH cohort while fasting glucose levels did not significantly differ from the healthy controls (see below; insulin up-regulated the expression and the activity of hepatic CYP2E1 in primary cultured rat hepatocytes). Another study reported a positive correlation between the severity of hepatic steatosis and hepatic CYP2E1 activity by the oral clearance of chlorzoxazone in morbidly obese patients with NASH [143]. These studies also showed that weight loss decreased hepatic CYP2E1 activity. In addition to the activation of CYP2E1, there are two other cytochrome P450s, namely CYP4A10 and 4A14, that have been suggested to play a role in animal studies (see above) [141]. CYP4A family is induced by PPARα that PPARα-deficient mice prevented the development of NASH.

Several investigators previously reported that increased mitochondrial and peroxisomal β-oxidation of fatty acids provided a large amount of ketone bodies to hepatic cytochromes. This induces cytochrome P450 gene expression and increases their protein level in the liver. However, this issue remains controversial with some recent observations. Woodcroft and colleagues used primary cultured rat hepatocytes in the absence of insulin to evaluate the effect of increased ketone bodies on the regulation of CYP2E1 expression, and showed no effect or even decreased CYP2E1 mRNA levels [199]. Moreover, these studies demonstrated that insulin decreased CYP2E1 mRNA and its protein levels by both suppressing CYP2E1 gene transcription and enhancing CYP2E1 mRNA degradation in an increased insulin concentration-dependent manner [199-201]. Similarly, De Waziers and colleagues previously had reported increased degradation of CYP2E1 mRNA by insulin in Fao rat hepatoma cells [202]. Additionally, Favreau and colleagues had demonstrated that administration of insulin reversed the increased expression of CYP2E1 in rats [132]. Wang and colleagues showed insulin supplementation in type 1 diabetics achieved close to normal CYP2E1 activities (similar to healthy controls) [196]. Furthermore, Woodcroft and colleagues reported that increased concentration of glucose in the medium might elevate CYP2E1 mRNA levels [199]. In parallel, Leclercq and colleagues previously had reported that dietary sugar restriction decreased CYP2E1 activity in human [203]. Lastly, Wang and colleagues showed an inverse relationship between chlorzoxazone area under the curve and fasting glucose levels [196]. These novel studies pointed out that insulin rather than ketone bodies, with or without glucose contribution, regulates the expression and activity of hepatic CYP2E1. With respect to the pathogenesis of NAFLD, insulin resistance and hyperglycemia are major metabolic hallmarks of NAFLD. These metabolic abnormalities increase hepatic CYP2E1 activity and subsequent prooxidant production in patients with NAFLD.

Moreover, Nieto and colleagues reported that CYP2E1-mediated oxidative stress induced collagen type 1 expression in rat HSC [204]. However, CYP2E1 expression was not demonstrated in human HSC [205]. It is also well-defined that CYPs both metabolize and activate carcinogens. It might be possible that increased production of activated carcinogens by CYPs might contribute to the development of liver cancer in patients with NASH.

Iron, Oxidant Stress and NASH

Iron can play a central role in promoting oxidant stress and this is proposed to be the mechanism of progressive liver disease in hemochromatosis. However, there is no convincing evidence for the role of iron in the pathogenesis of NASH [206-209]. Plasma and hepatic iron measurements, plasma ferritin levels, and genetic mutations of hemochromatosis gene (*HFE*) are the main parameters which have been used to investigate the contribution of iron in the pathogenesis of NASH. Recently, a large-population based study reported a correlation between elevated serum alanine aminotransferase levels and increased serum transferrin and iron concentrations [210]. Antioxidants were decreased as well. Another recent study evaluated 42 patients with carbohydrate-intolerance who had serum iron saturation lower than 50% and no C282Y and H63D *HFE* mutations [211].

After initial measurements, investigators induced iron depletion to a level of near-iron deficiency by phlebotomies. Interestingly, they observed improvements in both insulin sensitivity and serum alanine aminotransferase activity in some of the patients, indicating that iron may play a role not only in oxidant stress but also in the initial predisposing factor of insulin resistance. A recent prospective cohort study evaluated 263 patients with NASH for both hepatic and peripheral iron burden and *HFE* mutations (C282Y and H63D) and the investigators found that iron burden and *HFE* mutations did not significantly correlate with the hepatic fibrosis of NASH [26].

MITOCHONDRIAL DYSFUNCTION AND ATP DEPLETION

Mitochondria are the organelles primarily responsible for fatty acid β-oxidation and oxidative phosphorylation, the process responsible for the production of ATP. Mitochondria are also a source of a limited amount of ROS production under physiologic conditions (see above) [126,128]. Several observations including decreased mitochondrial enzyme activities and increased fat concentration of skeletal muscle cells in obese or diabetic patients have suggested mitochondrial dysfunction in these disorders. Such abnormalities may increase ROS production and promote both oxidative stress and lipid peroxidation within the hepatocyte. Mitochondrial dysfunction is frequently due to a combination of genetic abnormalities, physical inactivity, aging, lipotoxicity (free fatty acids), lipid peroxidation (mitochondrial DNA alterations), and TNF-α [118,126].

The hepatocyte is a cell rich in mitochondria and some studies have suggested that each hepatocyte contains approximately 800 mitochondria, although other investigators have suggested that mitochondria form an interconnected network and are thus difficult to enumerate [127,128,162]. Mitochondria contain their own genomic DNA located in the matrix and this DNA encodes a limited number of components of the MRC. The majority of mitochondrial proteins are encoded by nuclear DNA. Hepatic mitochondrial abnormalities have been identified in NAFLD, suggesting that mitochondria may be the source or target of injury and that ineffective mitochondrial function resulting in cellular ATP depletion may be important pathophysiological processes in NAFLD and NASH [212]

The presence of megamitochondria, or mitochondrial swelling, is a microscopically detectable structural abnormality of hepatocyte mitochondria found in a variety of liver diseases including NAFLD [21,213,214]. Crystalline inclusions within the mitochondrial matrix have been documented in patients with NASH by electron microscopy. The composition and function of these crystals remain to be established. The presence of megamitochondria might be related to MRC enzyme complex deficiencies or oxidative phosphorylation abnormalities of mitochondria. In one study, the presence of lipid peroxidation, demonstrated by 3-nitrotyrosine staining in liver specimens, was noted to a minor degree in normal livers and was marked in both fatty liver and NASH with significantly higher amount in NASH than in fatty liver [21]. The same study also showed that the abundance of megamitochondria with crystalline inclusions was increased in patients with NASH (nine of ten patients) compared to patients with steatosis alone (none of eight patients), hepatitis C (one of ten patients), and controls (none of six potential donors). Marked differences in mitochondrial inclusions within the same liver and cell to cell variability for this feature in patients with NASH were also noted [21,213,215]. Despite the correlation of mitochondrial abnormalities with NASH, another study of NASH patients reported that there was no correlation between the abundance of megamitochondria and the stage of NASH (stages 1 and 2 vs stages 3 and 4), zones of NASH (zone 1 vs zone 3), severity of lipid peroxidation (low vs high), and ballooning hepatocytes (0-1 vs 2-3) [214]. These studies have also found that two patients with NASH-associated cirrhosis lose their mitochondrial inclusions as well as other histologic features of NASH by the time their disease has progressed to cirrhosis [10,214,216]. Why this occurs has not been established.

Hepatic mitochondrial DNA levels and the protein products of the mitochondrial genes are also decreased in patients with NASH. Earlier studies reported normal activity of complex I and complex III in platelet-derived mitochondria of patients with NASH [213], although no defect in the MRC enzyme expression in the muscles of one NASH patient was reported [21]. However, later evidence showed that NASH was associated with decreased cytochrome c oxidase activity in the mitochondria. Finally, decreased hepatic activity of all MRC enzyme complexes by 30% to 50% of control activity (from complex 1 to complex 5) was reported in patients with NASH [217]. Impaired hepatic MRC function increases ROS production and if ROS production exceeds antioxidant capabilities, oxidative stress and injury, lipid peroxidation of macromolecules and cellular membranes, mitochondrial DNA damage, direct damage of several mitochondrial enzymes, and further MRC dysfunction with more prooxidant production are observed. A very recent study pointed out the relationship between long chain fatty acid oxidation abnormalities due to a mitochondrial trifunctional protein (MTP) defect and the development of both insulin resistance and hepatic steatosis in mice [218]. In addition to a MTP defect, aging was an important factor in the development of these disturbances. Mixed macro- and microvesicular steatosis due to β-oxidation defects in the mitochondria was the predominant type of steatosis in this study and CYP 2E1 expression was upregulated and levels of the antioxidant glutathione were decreased.

TNF-α, a cytokine implicated in NASH, diminishes hepatocyte mitochondrial permeability, blocks MRC electron flow, and eventually causes increased ROS production [126,167,217, 219]. A study recently demonstrated a significant correlation between increased circulating TNF-α levels and mitochondrial dysfunction in patients with NASH [217].

Mitochondrial uncoupling protein 2 (UCP2) is a mitochondrial inner membrane protein. It might regulate proton leak across the mitochondrial inner membrane, promote ATP depletion, and inversely regulate ROS production. Depletion of the energy (ATP) stores increases the susceptibility of hepatocytes to various injury [164] while decreased ROS production limits the hepatocyte injury. Thus, whether UCP2 is harmful or protective in the liver remains unestablished. Several studies demonstrated up-regulation of hepatic UCP2 expression in obese animals provided by genetically (*ob/ob*) or a high-fat diet [164,220-222]. UCP 2 might be responsible for hepatocellular injury in NAFLD, but a recent animal study, performed with UCP2 deficient mice, failed to show any protective or harmful effects of UCP2 in obesity induced fatty livers [223].

Carnitine and two CPTs (CPT-I and CPT-II) are required to transfer long-chain free fatty acids into the mitochondria for β-oxidation. Some investigators reported the role of carnitine deficiency in NAFLD development [224,225] while others observed normal hepatic content of total and free carnitine in patients with NASH [217]. CPT activities were also observed to be normal in patients with NASH [217].

FREE FATTY ACID TOXICITY

In addition to insulin resistance and hyperinsulinemia, obesity and type 2 diabetes mellitus are strongly associated with increased concentration of free fatty acids in the circulation [64,226,227]. Similar observations have been made in patients with NAFLD [1]. Fatty acids are involved in many important cellular events such as synthesis of cellular membranes, energy storage, and intracellular signaling pathways. However, chronically elevated free fatty acids have the capability to disturb diverse metabolic pathways and induce insulin resistance in many organ systems (see above, cellular mechanisms of insulin resistance) [107,228-233]. Fatty acids also interact with glucose metabolism. In addition to their metabolic effects, fatty acids could induce cellular apoptosis, also called as lipotoxicity, in two ways: direct toxicity and an indirect effect. One proposed mechanism of fatty acid toxicity in hepatocytes is that fatty acids induce translocation of Bax (which is a mitochondrial protein and a member of Bcl-2 family) to lysosomes and cause lysosomal destabilization which promotes the release of cathepsin B (ctsb, a specific lysosomal enzyme), from lysosomes to cytosol. Subsequently, a cathepsin B dependent process induces NF-κB activation and TNF-α overexpression in the liver [219]. TNF-α might further increase lysosomal destabilization and cathepsin B dependent hepatocyte apoptosis [104,234,235]. Then, cytochrome c release from the mitochondria with mitochondrial dysfunction may occur. Mitochondrial dysfunction causes energy depletion which activates proteolytic caspases and induces DNA fragmentation and chromatin condensation. Moreover, activated caspases cleave the Bcl-2 family proteins and cause further mitochondrial damage while activating DNases that produce DNA breaks [236-238]. NF-κB is a transcriptional factor and has both apoptotic and anti-apoptotic effect. In healthy hepatocytes, activation of NF-κB by TNF-α induces Bcl-2 synthesis which prevents the release of cytochrome c from the mitochondria and subsequent apoptosis [104,239]. Feldstein and colleagues demonstrated that genetically cathepsin B deficient or pharmacologically cathepsin B inactivated mice did not exhibit the development of fatty liver, liver injury, and insulin resistance in a dietary murine model [219]. Moreover, while cathepsin B was demonstrated in hepatocyte lysosomes of healthy control subjects, the majority of hepatocytes in patients with NAFLD showed diffuse distribution of cathepsin B in the cytosol, with a positive correlation with the stage of NASH.

Most recently, Ji and colleagues demonstrated hepatocyte apoptosis induced by the saturated fatty acid palmitic acid in rat hepatocytes [104]. The authors suggested that a mitochondria-mediated apoptosis pathway (intrinsic pathway), which includes two mitochondrial proteins such as Bax and Bcl-2, regulates this process. The authors observed a mild decrease in Bcl-2 levels and a marked increase in Bax levels. Bax induces and Bcl-2 inhibits hepatocyte apoptosis, and they work independently [104,240-242]. The Bcl-2/Bax ratio regulates the release of cytochrome c from the mitochondria and subsequent apoptosis. A significantly decreased Bcl-2/Bax ratio promoted apoptosis in HepG2 cells in these studies [104]. These studies also showed dose- and time-dependent inhibition of cellular growth in rat hepatocytes.

In addition to these mechanisms, there are two other possibilities: ceramide, synthesized de novo from fatty acids and a lipid signaling molecule, might promote apoptosis and elevated free fatty acids may increase oxidative stress and subsequently promote apoptosis [243].

ENDOGENOUS TOXINS: ENDOTOXIN AND GUT-DERIVED ETHANOL

The link between gut flora and liver disease was firmly established after the development of severe and sometimes fatal fatty liver disease in patients with morbid obesity following jejunoileal bypass operation [244]. Some of these patients required liver transplantation and some of the newly transplanted livers developed NASH. It was also observed that antibiotic administration, particularly metronidazole, or surgical removal of the blind loop improved hepatic abnormalities [245-247]. Subsequent observations also include a patient with jejunal diverticulosis and intestinal bacterial overgrowth that appeared to cause NASH [248].

Additional information regarding this process was obtained by animal studies. Investigators showed that *ob/ob* leptin deficient mice produce increased levels of breath ethanol compared to control animals and administration of nonabsorbable antibiotics decreased breath ethanol levels, implicating gut flora as a source of absorbed ethanol in mice [249], a finding not confirmed in humans. A small pilot study performed with obese female patients with NAFLD showed increased breath ethanol concentrations [250]. A subsequent study evaluated the relationship between small intestinal bacterial overgrowth and NASH by measuring a combined ^{14}C-D-xylose and lactulose breath test and correlating these with plasma TNF-α and endotoxin concentrations [251]. Additionally, intestinal permeability was assessed. This study found significantly increased blood TNF-α concentrations and small intestinal bacterial overgrowth in patients with NASH compared to sex and age matched controls. Intestinal permeability and serum endotoxin levels were not different between the groups. However, mean BMI and the prevalence of diabetes were higher in NASH group than controls in this study, suggesting an interplay between insulin resistance and gut-derived endotoxin to cause NASH. The same may be true for gut-derived ethanol as breath ethanol concentrations correlated with increased BMI in NASH patients [250]. The mechanisms underlying these interactions have not been established, but one explanation is increased ethanol and LPS production by bacteria in the small bowel disrupts mucosal integrity and increase intestinal permeability. Absorbed bacterial products may stimulate hepatocytes and Kupffer cells to produce ROS and inflammatory cytokines that contribute to insulin resistance, hepatocyte apoptosis, necroinflammation, and fibrosis. Limited clinical studies have tested this interaction and have found that antibiotics, probiotics, TNF-α receptor antagonism, and surgical elimination of blind loops improved some features of NASH in both animal models and humans [249,252-254].

ADIPOCYTOKINES

Adipocytokines, adipose tissue derived hormones and cytokines originating from adipose tissue, are often abnormally·expressed in patients with NASH and these abnormalities may play a role in pathogenesis of NASH [255-257]. It is now recognized that adipose tissue is not only a storage site for excess metabolic energy in the form of fat, it has also important endocrine and immunologic functions [42,258,259]. Adipose tissue releases a variety of adipocytokines, signaling proteins, fatty acids, and other bioactive lipids that regulate inflammation and metabolism in the liver and elsewhere in the body. Some of the important adipocytokines are TNF-α, IL-6, adiponectin, leptin, and resistin. These adipose tissue products regulate both glucose and lipid metabolisms and insulin sensitivity of the insulin target cells. Additionally, receptors for proinflammatory cytokines such as TNF-α and IL-6 are expressed on the surface of adipocytes indicating that adipocytes, like other insulin-sensitive cells respond to signaling by these mediators. Some adipocytokines such as TNF-α and IL-6 are also the products of macrophages within adipose tissue, a recent finding that suggests an inflammatory state with adipose tissue may regulate metabolism in adipocytes and, by implication, also in downstream tissues such as the liver [76,153]. Furthermore, preadipocytes under some conditions could exhibit phagocytic properties.

The anatomical location of adipose tissue plays an important role in provoking insulin resistance. Visceral, or intraabdominal, fat is lipolytically more active than subcutaneous fat and adipocytes of the former are less mature than those of the latter [260-264]. Visceral adipose tissue is a much more significant source for adipocytokines compared to subcutaneous fat, secreting more TNF-α and leptin while releasing more fatty acids than subcutaneous adipose tissue. In contrast, subcutaneous fat produces more adiponectin than visceral fat. Because of its anatomical location in the mesenteric circulation, visceral adipose tissue releases its adipocytokines and fatty acids directly to the liver via splanchics, a factor that may predispose to NAFLD and NASH. Indeed, removal of subcutaneous fat by liposuction did not improve metabolic abnormalities in one study [265].

Leptin

Leptin is a 16-kDa polypeptide synthesized and secreted by mature adipocytes under the control of *ob* gene [43,266,267]. Skeletal muscle cells and culture-activated HSC might also synthesize leptin and its expression is regulated by IL-1, TNF-α, and insulin [268,269]. Leptin is an endogenous anti-obesity cytokine-type hormone that inhibits food intake and increases energy expenditure at a central level. It has both peripheral actions via the long form of the leptin receptor and central actions via the sympathetic nervous system. The hypothalamus is one of the important sites of leptin effects [270]. Leptin binds the transmembrane leptin receptor Ob-R and Ob-Rb, a long-form leptin receptor, can activate the Janus kinase (JAK)/STAT pathway and phosphorylates STAT proteins [271-274] to induce the transcription of TGF-β1 and procollagen genes. Similarly, leptin causes phosphorylation of STAT-3 in cultured hepatic stellate cells, the cells responsible for fibrogenesis and cirrhosis. However, there is currently no consensus regarding the contribution of leptin to the liver injury and fibrosis [26,168,269,274-280].

As might be expected based on the biological effects of leptin, complete leptin deficient *ob/ob* mice exhibit hyperphagia, obesity, and diabetes caused by a natural homozygous mutation of the *ob* gene [270]. Exogenous leptin administration improved these abnormalities and reduced adipose tissue mass in *ob/ob* mice [43,281-283]. In fact, the beneficial effects of leptin on hyperglycemia and hyperinsulinemia were found with leptin doses which did not induce weight loss [43]. Although leptin may improve insulin sensitivity, the mechanism of this action is not clearly understood. Subjects with generalized lipodystrophy have decreased or absent adipose tissue and low plasma levels of its product, leptin. Loss of adipose tissue causes ectopic adipogenesis such as in the liver and induces insulin resistance in these organs by disturbing downstream insulin signaling. Exogenous leptin administration [284] or implantation of adipose tissue from wild-type mice to mice with generalized lipodystrophy [285] improved metabolic abnormalities such as insulin sensitivity. Improvements in the surgical group were observed after the enlargement and maturation of transplanted adipose tissue.

Leptin also has the ability to regulate immunologic functions such as stimulation of monocytes and induction of TNF-α secretion [176,286-291]. Additionally, leptin might cause oxidative stress, and proinflammatory and profibrogenic processes in the liver. Antisteatotic effects of leptin have been demonstrated in rodents [168,292] while some investigators reported a positive correlation between plasma leptin levels and hepatic steatosis in NASH patients [168]. In contrast, no correlation between serum leptin levels and steatosis, inflammation, ballooning cells, and Mallory bodies was reported [280]. Most recently, Javor and colleagues showed that exogenous leptin administration had no effect on fibrosis stage of NASH patients with severe lipodystrophy. However, the biopsy interval may have been too short to identify differences in this study as the mean duration was only 6.6 months [293].

Patients with absolute leptin deficiency due to a mutation of leptin gene are reported rarely [294]. These patients are morbidly obese and show both insulin resistance and hepatic steatosis. Recombinant methionyl human leptin (r-metHuLeptin) replacement therapy improved NASH activity scores, hepatic steatosis, aminotransferase levels, high triglycerides, fasting glucose levels, insulin resistance, and normalized body weight in leptin deficient, lipodystrophic human subjects [291,293]. This benefit might be related with the inhibition of neuropeptide Y and agouti-related protein synthesis and secretion in the hypothalamus. Other possibilities might be the activation of fatty acid oxidation enzymes, inhibition of lipogenic enzymes, induction of hepatic and adipose tissue PPAR-γ coactivator 1α expression, and activation of PPARα and AMP-activated protein kinase. Leptin might also regulate mitochondrial functions. It was reported that leptin reduced fat content in adipocytes and increased the number of mitochondria while leptin deficiency caused increased fat accumulation in adipocytes and functional deficiencies in the mitochondria [293].

Mutations and truncated leptin receptors have also been reported in humans [43,295]. These patients are obese due to the impaired leptin action. The presence of leptin resistance is also caused by abnormalities of intracellular signaling pathways of leptin. Most obese humans have increased plasma leptin levels which are correlated with adipose tissue mass [296-299]. Weight loss decreased both circulating leptin and inflammation markers [300,301].

Adiponectin

Adiponectin is a large 30 kDa polypeptide hormone (ACRP30) secreted by adipocytes. It has antilipogenic and anti-inflammatory effects [30,257,302-304].

Most evidence suggests that adiponectin is a necessary component of normal insulin action and improves insulin sensitivity by enhancing intracellular insulin signaling [169,305-307], although the adiponectin knockout mice may have normal insulin signaling and glucose tolerance [308]. An interesting relationship has emerged between TNF-α and adiponectin in which each down-regulates the expression and activity of the other [309-311].

At the cellular level, adiponectin induces β-oxidation of fatty acids and decreases muscle steatosis. Adiponectin decreases fatty acid content of the liver and increases hepatic insulin sensitivity by decreasing both plasma free fatty acid uptake and de novo synthesis of fatty acids and by increasing both mitochondrial β-oxidation of fatty acids and triglyceride export [302,312,313]. These effects reduce triglyceride content and glucose output of the liver. Adiponectin also may activate AMP-activated protein kinase and directly stimulate glucose uptake in both adipocytes and muscle cells. In addition to these effects, adiponectin may have anti-inflammatory properties such as inhibition of both phagocytic activity and TNF-α production of macrophages [314,315].

There is an inverse relationship between adiponectin mRNA expression and adipose tissue mass in both mice and humans. Plasma levels of adiponectin were also found to be inversely related to the adipose tissue mass and degree of insulin resistance in human subjects [316-318]. A study performed in Pima Indians showed that increased plasma adiponectin levels strongly correlated with a decreased risk of developing type 2 diabetes mellitus, independent of the presence of obesity [319]. Plasma adiponectin levels are inversely correlated with hyperinsulinemia and insulin resistance. This inverse relationship is less marked with increased adipose tissue mass. In addition to an increase in inflammatory response, adiponectin knockout mice also have high plasma levels of TNF-α and severe insulin resistance [169,305]. As might be expected, lipoatrophic mice that lack normal adipose tissue show decreased plasma adiponectin levels, as well as leptin deficiency and insulin resistance. These abnormalities could be reversed with the adiponectin administration.

Leptin-deficient *ob/ob* mice have reduced adiponectin concentrations and adiponectin treatment improved hepatomegaly and steatosis and decreased elevated serum aminotransferases and inflammation of the liver by inhibiting hepatic TNF-α production and fatty acid synthesis, and increasing fatty acid oxidation [170]. Adiponectin administration prevented hepatic fibrosis in wild-type mice treated with carbon tetrachloride. Moreover, the same study also demonstrated aggravated liver fibrosis in adiponectin knockout mice treated with carbon tetrachloride. Although patients with NASH have excess visceral fat, circulating adiponectin concentrations were found decreased independent of insulin resistance [171,320,321]. An association between reduced adiponectin levels and more extensive hepatic necroinflammation was also demonstrated [171]. Two adiponectin receptors, defined as AdipoR1 and AdipoR2, are expressed mainly in skeletal muscle and liver, respectively [302]. AdipoR1 has a high affinity for circulating globular adiponectin (gAd) while AdipoR2 has an intermediate affinity for both forms of adiponectin, full-length ligand and gAd. The levels of hepatic AdipoR2 mRNA expression in patients with NASH is uncertain because of conflicting data [320,321]. Thus, it remains unclear whether decreased hepatic Adipo R2 is an adaptive mechanism against decreased circulating adiponectin concentrations in patients with NASH.

TNF-α

TNF-α is a proinflammatory cytokine primarily synthesized and secreted by adipose tissue in the absence of malignancy or infection [30,43,322,323]. In addition to inflammation, TNF-α is involved in cell proliferation, differentiation, and apoptosis. Increased TNF-α production has been found in obesity with insulin resistance in both animal models and human subjects [154,322-328] while TNF-α levels decreased after weight lost [322,323]. Moreover, plasma TNF-α levels were reported to be elevated in both NAFLD and NASH patients [251,329] and TNF-α antibody infusions improved hepatic steatosis in ob/ob mice [254]. TNF-α is expressed as a cell surface transmembrane protein and can act in both autocrine and paracrine manners. TNF-α induces lipolysis and inhibits adipogenesis via TNF-R1, the ERK 1/2 pathway, and inhibition of PPAR-γ and lipogenesis [330-332] and it plays a major role in the pathogenesis of insulin resistance in both rodents and humans [150,322,333]. Overexpression of adipose tissue TNF-α mRNA and increased plasma TNF-α levels correlate with increased adipose tissue mass [322,323,334]. At the level of adipose tissue, TNF-α may induce insulin resistance by accelerating peripheral lipolysis with increased release of fatty acids, reducing adiponectin synthesis, and down-regulating the membrane expression of the GLUT4 glucose transporter [45,46,335]. In addition, TNF-α may inhibit lipoprotein lipase activity, reduce the expression of free fatty acid transporters, and decrease the expression of lipogenic enzymes in adipose tissue [323]. TNF-α might induce apoptosis of both preadipocytes and adipocytes.

It was also shown that treatment with insulin sensitizing agents decreased TNF-α concentrations and improved NASH features in both animal models and humans [215,329,336-339].

IL-6

IL-6 is a circulating proinflammatory cytokine that plays a role in insulin resistance [43,304,340-342]. It is primarily secreted by visceral adipocytes and binds to transmembrane receptors to initiate a signal transduction cascade leading to impaired insulin signal transduction via induction of SOCS-3 [343]. Clinical studies have established that plasma IL-6 levels are positively correlated with increased adipose tissue and insulin resistance [333,344,345]. Moreover, plasma and adipose tissue levels of IL-6 are decreased by weight loss [334]. Administration of IL-6 to healthy volunteers induces dose-dependent increases in blood glucose. IL-6 may also increase plasma free fatty acid levels due to its effects on increasing insulin resistance and decreasing adiponectin secretion.

Resistin

Resistin is an adipocytokine first identified in mice that is produced and released by mature adipocytes. In contrast, immune cells rather than adipocytes might be the major producer of resistin in humans [43,346,347]. Its expression is induced during adipocyte differentiation. Its role in insulin resistance is not clear in humans whereas it causes insulin resistance in mice. High resistin levels in the plasma were observed in both genetic (*ob/ob* and *db/db*) and diet-induced animal models of obesity [348]. Administration of resistin diminished glucose tolerance and insulin action in normal mice and, after the blocking of resistin effects, plasma glucose and insulin levels were decreased in insulin resistant *ob/ob* mice [349]. Whether these finding will be confirmed in humans is not certain.

Regulation of Hepatic Immunity and Increased Sensitivity to Hepatocellular Injury

As regulation of inflammation has become increasing recognized as a central modulator insulin sensitivity, attention has focused on components of innate and cellular immunity [175,350-352]. NKT cells are an important source of proinflammatory cytokines and specific depletion of hepatic NKT cells with consequent proinflammatory cytokine polarization of liver cytokine production exacerbated endotoxin-induced hepatic injury in the leptin deficient *ob/ob* mice [350]. IL-15 administration significantly increased the number of total and liver specific NKT cells, despite persistent leptin deficiency [175]. Additionally, noradrenaline treated *ob/ob* mice showed near normal to normal numbers of hepatic NKT cells and improved the balance between hepatic Th-1 and Th-2 cytokine productions, despite persistent leptin deficiency. These improvements resulted in activation of fibrogenesis in the livers of *ob/ob* mice [175]. Similarly, liver selective NKT cell deficiency and cytokine polarization in the fatty livers of wild-type mice fed with high fat or high sucrose or both had the same effect [353]. In normal biology, NKT cells move to and accumulate in the liver from the thymus. These cells regulate hepatic Th-1 and Th-2 cytokine production (proinflammatory and anti-inflammatory cytokines, respectively) by T cells, NKT cells, and other mononuclear cells in the liver. The selective depletion of hepatic NKT cells might be due to the increased NKT cell apoptosis; induction of fatty liver of dietary induced obese mice promotes hepatic Th-1 cytokine polarization and increased production of both TNF-α and INF-γ, the latter also being increased in the serum [353]. Proposed mechanisms for specific NKT depletion in the liver are decreased rates of NKT recruitment to the liver, decreased hepatic development of NKT cells, increased loss of NKT, or emigration from the liver, and surface markers loss identifying cells as NKT, or any combination of these effects [354]. After endotoxin treatment, inflammation, necrosis, and the concentration of serum liver enzymes as liver inflammation markers were increased significantly [353].

HEPATOCYTE APOPTOSIS IN NAFLD

Apoptosis, or programmed cell death, is a reflection of normal cell turnover [238]. In the liver, turnover is normally slow and apoptotic cells are relatively rare. Hepatocyte apoptosis was observed more frequently in NASH patients compared to subjects with steatosis alone or control [355]. Fas, which is a death receptor, a surface glycoprotein and a member of TNF receptor family, and caspase activation are two common mediators of hepatocyte apoptosis [238,355-357]. Increased caspase activation and strongly upregulated Fas expression were noted in patients with NASH [355]. Additionally, a positive relationship between the abundance of hepatocyte apoptosis, demonstrated by TUNEL-positive cells histologically, and both the grade and stage of NASH was found, suggesting that apoptosis is not entirely silent with respect to inflammation, fibrogenesis, and even in the development of cirrhosis [238,355,357]. Oxidative stress is a contributor to hepatocyte apoptosis and ROS increase TNF-α and Fas ligand expression on hepatocytes [234,357,358]. Oxidative stress degrades IκB which is the inhibitor of NF-κB. Activated NF-κB has the capability to induce or inhibit apoptotic events in the hepatocytes (see above). Indeed, NF-κB is a regulator of inflammatory cytokine expression, Bcl-2 family and caspase functions. Hepatic NF-κB expression is increased in patients with NASH [357]. Also, increased Fas expression on the surface of lipid laden mouse (fed a high caloric diet) hepatocytes has been shown [356]. In addition to increased TNF-α secretion, expression of TNF receptor 1 (TNF-R1), a death receptor, was upregulated in patients with NASH [355]. It was recently reported that hepatocyte injury and death in patients with NASH is also associated with increased TNF-R1 mediated apoptosis [238]

It may be that hepatocytes in patients with NASH are more sensitized to death ligands (Fas and TNF-α) due to increased death receptor (Fas and TNF-R1) expression on the surface of these hepatocytes. This could promote apoptosis of hepatocytes via extrinsic stimuli in NASH (death receptor pathway or extrinsic pathway). These events eventually cause cytochrome c release from mitochondria, activation of caspases, mitochondrial dysfunction and other apoptotic events (see above).

Fatty acids-induced hepatocyte apoptosis is discussed previously (see above; free fatty acid toxicity).

Chapter 4

HEPATIC FIBROGENESIS IN NASH

ROLE OF STELLATE CELLS AND CYTOKINES IN HEPATIC FIBROGENESIS

HSC are the main collagen producing cells in the liver and are responsible for fibrosis [359-362]. After activation, HSC proliferate and transform into myofibroblast like cells that lose their retinoid droplets and express α-smooth muscle actin (αSMA). Activated HSC express myogenic markers such as c-myb and myocyte enhancer factor-2, exhibit proinflammatory and profibrogenic properties, migrate and secrete extracellular matrix components (ECM) such as collagen, and regulate the degradation of ECM. Activation of HSC is the crucial step in liver fibrogenesis in a process regulated by autocrine and paracrine factors.

A study of NAFLD patients (16 patients with steatosis alone and 60 patients with NASH) demonstrated that activation of HSC was positive in almost all cases and markedly in two thirds of patients and it was correlated with the degree and location of hepatic fibrosis [359]. Interestingly, this study showed no relationship between the activation of HSC and the severity of necroinflammation and steatosis or stainable iron, but in general, both fibrosis and activated HSC were commonly observed in zone 3 which is also the most affected zone in NASH. HSC activation and upregulation of profibrogenic genes (e.g., collagen α1, and TIMP-1 and -2) were also observed in rats on a high-fat, MCD diet [363]. Additionally, lipid peroxidation associated inflammation and HSC activation with increased TGFβ1 mRNA expression in MCD steatohepatitis models were reported [186,363].

Genetic and environmental factors may affect the development of liver fibrosis in NAFLD. While the genetic factors remain to be elucidated, age, severity of obesity, presence of diabetes, and hyperglycemia are the major non-genetic factors. Elevated plasma glucose, free fatty acids and adipocytokines, which are the important players of NAFLD pathogenesis, activate both Kupffer cells and HSC and eventually stimulate fibrogenesis. Paradis and colleagues investigated the relationship between metabolic factors (hyperglycemia and insulin resistance) and connective tissue growth factor (CTGF), a cytokine that plays a role in the development of liver fibrogenesis, both in vivo in both human NASH and diabetic and obese rats, and in vitro on HSC [364]. In these studies, hepatic CTGF mRNA was overexpressed in all NASH subjects while hepatic CTGF mRNA and its protein were upregulated in *fa/fa* rats (obese and diabetic) compared with their lean littermates. The same group also demonstrated upregulation of both CTGF mRNA and its protein in HSC after exposure to high concentrations of either glucose or insulin. These results correlate with clinical NASH studies and with the pathogenesis of NAFLD. A study demonstrated that insulin resistance is independently associated with the degree of fibrosis in patients with NASH [26] and another study of overweight patients reported that hyperglycemia is a negative prognostic factor in the evolution of NASH towards fibrosis [365]. These effects of glucose and insulin appeared to be independent of TGF-β.

Oxidative stress may also participate in the activation of HSC and the development of fibrosis in NAFLD [186,363,366-368]. The intracellular NADPH oxidase pathway produces ROS and the disruption of NADPH oxidase protected mice from developing severe liver injury. Lipid peroxidation products and leptin also enhance the production of both TGF-β and collagen.

The role of leptin in fibrogenesis remains to be determined despite many efforts to date [168,175,191,293,369]. Initial studies, performed with *ob/ob*, genetically leptin deficient mice, showed that leptin critically regulates liver fibrogenesis [274,277,370,371]. The most probable mechanism for leptin effects is activation of the PI3-K pathway [274]. A direct effect of leptin on HSC in culture has also been reported [372]. Administration of leptin stimulated HSC to upregulate α2 (I) collagen gene expression. Leptin interferes with the production of cytokines (Th-2) such as IL-10 [175] and the balance between proinflammatory Th-1 and profibrogenic Th-2 cytokines regulates fibrogenesis in the liver. Administration of leptin improved Th-2 cytokines and the fibrogenic response of liver in leptin deficient mice. This is an example of an indirect leptin effect on fibrogenesis. The same group also pointed out the relation between NKT cells, which regulate the production of liver cytokines, and leptin. Leptin administration increased the viability and reduced the increased apoptosis rates of NKT cells in leptin deficient *ob/ob* mice. Additionally, the same group showed that norepinephrine, which is a leptin inducible factor, promotes liver fibrosis (see above). A recently performed study of human NAFLD and leptin reported that increased leptin levels in NASH patients simply reflect both increased age and insulin concentrations in the plasma and are not related with the advanced stages of NASH [280].

Angiotensin II, a vasoactive cytokine, plays an important role in liver fibrogenesis [362,373]. Angiotensin II expression is upregulated in the chronically injured liver and induces both hepatic inflammation and fibrogenic actions. It was also shown that decreased renin-angiotensin system activation markedly improved experimentally developed liver fibrosis. An angiotensin II receptor antagonist, losartan, has been used in hypertensive patients with NASH for 48 weeks and it decreased both plasma TGF-β1 and aminotransferase levels [374]. Additionally, the grade of hepatic necroinflammation, stage of fibrosis, and the amount of iron deposition in the liver were decreased in some subjects.

HEPATOCELLULAR CARCINOMA

HCC is a late complication in the course of NAFLD that has progressed to cirrhosis [375-381]. Because epidemiologic data attributes the majority of cases of cryptogenic cirrhosis to prior NASH, the hepatocellular carcinoma found to occur in cryptogenic cirrhosis is now also associated with NASH as a predisposing risk [9,14,15,216,382,383]. For unexplained reasons, the characteristic histopathological features of NASH often disappear as the disease progresses to cirrhosis, resulting in an absence of diagnostic criteria in many patients with cryptogenic cirrhosis. The reported the incidence of NASH-associated HCC has been variably reported as 1.73% [9,216], 6.9% [15], 7.31% [378], 13% [382], and 27% [14] among the NASH patients with or without cirrhosis, with or without obesity. Diabetes increases the incidence of HCC by 1.3-2.4 -fold while viral hepatitis causes 13-19 fold increase in the risk of HCC [380]. Additionally, patients with NASH-associated HCC may be slightly older than patients with HCC due to other causes such as alcohol or viral hepatitis [14,15,380,384].

As opposed to human NASH-associated HCC, animal models of HCC can occur in non-cirrhotic livers [60]. It was also reported that increased TNF-α activity might be a necessary component for HCC development besides insulin resistance and fatty liver. Pten is a tumor suppresser gene which is decreased or is absent in some of the primary hepatoma patients. Investigators reported that hepatocytes of mice with hepatocyte specific Pten null mutation showed adipogenic-like transformation, and activated genes of both lipogenesis and fatty acid β-oxidation. The livers of these mice showed a similar histology to human NAFLD and NASH, and then progressed to liver cell adenoma and HCC over time [385]. However, in contrast to human NASH pathogenesis, insulin sensitivity of these mice was increased. Investigators concluded that Pten/PI3K pathways might be involved in the pathogenesis of the development of NASH-associated HCC [385]. An animal model study with hereditary fatty liver showed high incidence of spontaneous development of HCC in non-obese Shionogi mice after one year [386]. Male mice were affected more frequently and earlier than female mice in this study. These mice exhibited progression of disease from fatty liver to NASH, NASH-associated cirrhosis and eventually HCC. However, fld and jvs mice with hereditary fatty liver did not progress to HCC. Similarly, aromatase deficient mice did not develop HCC despite the severe fatty liver [387].

Currently, proposed mechanisms for the transformation from NASH to NASH-associated HCC are severe and cumulative oxidative stress to the hepatocytes, production of damaged DNA, defective or inhibited DNA repair systems, chronic continued hepatocyte injury and inflammatory infiltration, impaired antioxidant systems, and increased cell cycle of hepatocytes. Animal and human studies have also indicated that a connection between age, gender and the disease might be possible.

Chapter 5

PATHOPHYSIOLOGY OF THE PATHOLOGICAL FEATURES OF NASH

NAFLD is a clinicopathologic diagnosis. We should bear in mind that the pathogenesis of NASH is accompanied with the histological changes of NASH (Table 3). As mentioned earlier, genetic tendencies and environmental factors cause obesity and insulin resistance. In this background, different mechanisms such as insulin resistance and hyperinsulinemia, increased free fatty acids in the circulation and their toxicity, disturbed production of adipocytokines, increased oxidative stress, iron overload, and mitochondrial dysfunctions induce the development of NAFLD and NASH. Hepatic steatosis is the most frequent and initially observed morphological feature of these processes. Steatosis, inflammation, glycogen nuclei, lipogranulomas, ballooning of hepatocytes, Mallory bodies, and fibrosis are the major features of NAFLD.

Table 3. Histopathologic abnormalities in NASH.

- Steatosis
- Mixed lobular inflammation
- Hepatocyte ballooning with or without Mallory's hyaline
- Variable perisinusoidal fibrosis

MICROVESICULAR AND MACROVESICULAR STEATOSIS

Increased accumulation of triglycerides as fat droplets within the cytoplasm of hepatocytes is the first step in the development of steatosis. Although two different types of lipid vacuoles as microvesicular and macrovesicular have been identified depending on the size of vacuoles (< 1 micron or vacuoles smaller than the hepatocyte nucleus and > 1 micron in diameter, respectively), the most frequent type found in NAFLD is macrovesicular [388-393]. Mixed type lipid vacuoles are reported as well. Macrovesicular steatosis is typically characterized by a single fat droplet within the cytoplasm of the hepatocyte causing the displacement of the nucleus. In contrast, small lipid droplets and a centrally located nucleus characterize microvesicular steatosis. The observation of microvesicular fat alone is often indicative of causes other than typical NAFLD, particularly rapidly progressive diseases such as acute fatty liver of pregnancy and Reye's syndrome [394].

There may be differences in the causative factors or the development mechanisms between these two types of steatosis. Compared to macrovesicular steatosis, microvesicular steatosis is frequently reported as a consequence of severe mitochondrial injury or dysfunction [392,395,396]. This kind of pathology may be genetic such as MTP deficiency, or acquired due to toxins or drugs such as valproic acid and high doses of tetracycline. One possibility is that mitochondrial injury and dysfunction are not so severe in patients with NAFLD as to stimulate the development of microvesicular steatosis. However, as we mentioned earlier, the presence of mixed macro- and micro- steatosis in some NAFLD biopsies is not unusual. An explanation for this observation might be that mitochondrial injury and dysfunction is substantial enough to stimulate microvesicular development in addition to macrovesicular development, but not so severe as to stimulate a microvesicular development alone. Another possibility is that microvesicular development might develop in a shorter time than that required for macrovesicular development. This idea is supported by the association of acute toxin exposure in the development of microvesicular steatosis. However, we have no information whether such small lipid vacuoles reflect newly synthesized fat droplets, or if the aggregation of micro lipid vacuoles produces macro sized lipid vacuoles over time.

INFLAMMATION

Proinflammatory cytokines, oxidative stress and lipid peroxidation products appear to promote inflammatory infiltration in NASH [21,184, 187,191,397,398]. However, it remains unestablished whether inflammation is primary due to increased proinflammatory cytokines or secondary to the oxidative stress or both. Mixed lobular inflammation, which includes small numbers of polymorphonuclear leukocytes, lymphocytes, and macrophages, is a typical finding in NASH [392,396]. This type of inflammation is usually mild. In contrast, portal inflammation is usually not predominant in adult NASH patients whereas it can be seen in children [399].

GLYCOGEN NUCLEI

Glycogen nuclei, or glycogenated hepatocyte nuclei, are complex carbohydrate deposits of the hepatocyte nuclei found in a variety of disorders including diabetes, Wilson's disease and NAFLD [392,400]. They are one of the important pathological changes in diabetics or obese patients. The presence of glycogen nuclei is reported to be a reliable marker for distinguishing diabetics from non-diabetics. Although these are not specific findings or reliable markers for the etiology of NASH, they are commonly seen in diabetic NASH patients (up to 100%) [392,401].

LIPOGRANULOMAS

Lipogranulomas are common, seen in up to 82% of patients, but are not specific histologic findings of NASH patients [392,396]. Phagocytic consumption of lipid laden hepatocytes is the main reason of lipogranuloma development. As a consequence, small fat cysts can develop which promote inflammation and eventually lipogranuloma formation. A well-established lipogranuloma contains a central fat vacuole, macrophages, occasional giant cells, and sometimes lymphocytes and eosinophils.

HEPATOCELLULAR BALLOONING

Ballooned hepatocytes and Mallory bodies are two pathological features described as indicators of ongoing necroinflammation, and are used for grading necroinflammation and as predictors of further stages [402]. At the present time, we have no information whether they are adaptive (physiological), or degenerative (pathological) features of hepatocytes. Only one study carried out in patients with NAFLD has investigated the nature of ballooning hepatocytes to date [162]. This study reported the similarity between the lipid laden hepatocytes and adipose tissue cells. Additionally, few ballooned hepatocytes which had the evidence of hepatocyte degeneration, apoptosis, and necrosis were reported.

MALLORY BODIES AND STRESS PROTEINS

Stress proteins such as protein p62, HSP 27, and HSP 70 bind other abnormal proteins and form intermediate misfolded proteins [403-405]. Under normal conditions, the ubiquitin-proteasome pathway eliminates these harmful products. When this protective system fails, abnormal cytokeratins accumulate along with p62, HSP 27, HSP 70, ubiquitinated proteins and ropy structures recognized as Mallory bodies develop within ballooned hepatocytes. There are two possible ways for this pathway to fail: production rate of these misfolded proteins that exceeds the capacity of protective systems or inhibition of the protective pathways. The mechanisms of Mallory body formation in humans have not been fully understood yet. Misfolded proteins such as HSPs and other abnormal proteins are the response of hepatocytes to stressors and appear to be degenerative rather than adaptive.

GENETIC SUSCEPTIBILITY TO NASH AND THE BASIS OF NASH-PATHOPHYSIOLOGY

In addition to environmental factors, some evidence discussed previously pointed out genetic susceptibility to both development and progression of NASH. For example, although the majority of patients with insulin resistance or metabolic syndrome develop steatosis alone (NAFLD), only a minor group of these subjects progress to advanced stages of NASH. The progression rate of fibrosis is also reported to be variable among NASH patients [17,406-408]. Moreover, both obesity and type 2 diabetes mellitus which have well-established risks of inheritance [409] and are closely associated with NASH. NASH-associated cirrhosis and HCC were also more prevalent among the patients with type 2 diabetes mellitus with or without obesity [10,11,15,390]. Additionally, familial forms of NASH related with lipodystrophy have been reported [410]. Lastly, clustering of both cryptogenic cirrhosis and NASH were reported in kindreds of patients with NASH, besides the familial aggregation of insulin resistance in patients with NASH [411].

NASH Prevalence in Different Racial and Ethnic Groups

A few recently performed epidemiologic studies provided important evidence regarding genetic risks for NASH [8,412-415]. Although two well-known major risk factors of NASH, obesity and type 2 diabetes mellitus, are more prevalent among African Americans than in Caucasians and Hispanics, epidemiologic studies pointed out significant ethnic and racial variations in the prevalence of hepatic steatosis, NASH, and NASH-associated cirrhosis among these different racial and ethnic groups. Caldwell and colleagues evaluated patients with NASH (159 patients) or cyptogenic cirrhosis (206 patients) and demonstrated only one NASH case and only two cryptogenic cirrhosis cases among African Americans [412]. In contrast, the same study showed overrepresentation of both hepatitis C and hepatic sarcoidosis among African Americans. Browning and colleagues evaluated patients with cryptogenic cirrhosis and reported that cryptogenic cirrhosis-associated with obesity and diabetes is more prevalent among Hispanics and Caucasians, but rare among African Americans [413]. Browning and colleagues also evaluated the impact of ethnicity on the prevalence of hepatic steatosis in a separate study performed with a large, multi-ethnic, population-based sample [8]. Similar to the previously performed two studies [412,413], the authors reported the prevalence of hepatic steatosis to be significantly lower in African Americans than in both Hispanics and Caucasians. Weston and colleagues recently performed a cross-sectional study with newly diagnosed patients with chronic liver disease [414]. The authors reported overrepresentation of Hispanics with NAFLD. It appears that particularly Hispanics with NAFLD may progress to both NASH and cirrhosis more frequently than either blacks or whites. Lastly, Solga and colleagues prospectively evaluated 237 morbidly obese patients undergone bariatric surgery and compared hepatic histopathology features of African Americans with the hepatic histopathology of Caucasians [415]. The authors reported that NAFLD is more common and highly severe among Caucasians. In contrast, African Americans are less likely to have severe NAFLD histopathology. Moreover, Solga and colleagues proposed an African American race-related protection from obesity related liver disease. However, this race-related protection does not cover other chronic liver diseases, such as hepatitis C and hepatic sarcoidosis. Xanthakos and colleagues recently evaluated the prevalence of hepatic steatosis in a population-based cohort of young adult females (aged 24 to 27 years) by magnetic resonance imaging [416]. Of the 281 patients, 56% were African Americans and 44% were white. Although African Americans were significantly more obese and had higher mean leptin and insulin levels and waist circumferences than whites, the prevalence of hepatic steatosis was lower in African Americans than whites. The same study also showed that significant hepatic steatosis was not very prevalent in young adult females despite 42% obesity, 34% central obesity, and 41% elevated fasting insulin in this cohort. These results might reflect differences in the genetic susceptibility of different racial and ethnic groups to both development and progression of NASH.

NAFLD and Genes Associated with Lipid and Glucose Metabolism, Oxidant and Anti-Oxidant Systems, and Proinflammatory Cytokines

Insulin resistance, increased oxidant mediators, decreased antioxidants, and increased production of proinflammatory cytokines are the hallmarks of the pathogenesis of NASH. Thus, investigators evaluated the genes involved in lipid and glucose metabolism, oxidant and antioxidant systems, and the regulation of proinflammatory cytokines [167,207,417-420].

Sreekumar and colleagues investigated hepatic gene expression in patients with NASH-associated cirrhosis, with a particular emphasis on genetic evidence of both insulin resistance and mitochondrial dysfunction, and compared these results with those of healthy subjects and patients with cirrhosis due to hepatitis C or primary biliary cirrhosis [419]. The authors reported sixteen genes which were uniquely and differentially expressed in cirrhotic-NASH patients. Some of the under-expressed genes are important for free fatty acid metabolism (long chain acyl-CoA synthetase and mitochondrial 3-oxoacyl-Co A thiolase) or important for glucose metabolism (glucose-6-phosphatase and alcohol dehydrogenase). Other under-expressed genes are important for maintaining the mitochondrial functions such as copper-zinc superoxide dismutase, aldehyde oxidase and catalase (important for DNA repair and metabolism). Some of the overexpressed genes are involved in the diminished insulin sensitivity. Additionally, upregulated expression of insulin-like growth factor binding protein-1 and down-regulated expression of apoB 100 were reported while expression of superoxide dismutase-1 (SOD-1) which is involved in scavenging of ROS was found to be decreased in NASH patients. These observations also suggest that impaired repair and metabolism of DNA with increased oxidative mediators and decreased antioxidants might be the cause of mitochondrial DNA mutation and deletion in patients with NASH. Decreased synthesis of apoB 100 in NASH patients, reported previously by the same study group, correlated with the down-regulated expression of hepatic apoB 100. The authors also reported over-expression of some inflammation markers such as hepatocyte-derived fibrinogen-related protein 1, complement component C3, and α-1 antitrypsin in cirrhotic-NASH patients. This evidence further suggests the possibility of a genetic predisposition to NASH.

In another study, Younossi and colleagues studied 91 morbidly obese patients with NAFLD undergone bariatric surgery (27 patients had biopsy-proven NASH) and compared these patients with obese controls [420]. The authors demonstrated differential expression of several hepatic genes and proteins. Most importantly, the authors observed overall down-regulation of phase 2 detoxification enzymes which are important components of the cellular defense system against oxidative stress, such as glutathione S-transferase and cytosolic sulfotransferase isoform 1A2 among three groups (steatosis alone, steatosis and non-specific inflammation, and NASH) and in patients with more advanced stages of NASH, respectively. Increased expression of genes associated with the activation of HSC and fibrogenesis was also reported. These findings were correlated with the proposed mechanisms for the pathophysiology of NASH. Several investigators have also pointed out polymorphisms of the gene sequences encoding the TNF-α promoter, MTP, MTTP, SOD-2, CYP2E1, and apoB 100 may play a role in the pathogenesis of NAFLD [124,125,167,417,418,421].

Chapter 6

SUMMARY

NAFLD describes a spectrum of liver abnormalities from benign steatosis to NASH which is characterized by chronic and progressive liver pathology. Although the progression rate of NASH is most likely slower than the other types of liver disease, the prevalence of NASH and its consequences such as cirrhosis and HCC are increasing throughout the world. Currently, our understanding regarding NASH is that adipocytes accumulate excess energy as fat droplets and respond with dysregulated production of adipocytokines. Increased free fatty acids, predominantly due to peripheral lipolysis and proinflammatory cytokines, interfere with insulin signaling mechanisms to cause both local and peripheral insulin resistance. In addition to increased plasma free fatty acids that are taken up by the liver, insulin resistance, elevated plasma insulin, and elevated glucose levels activate de novo fatty acid and triglyceride synthesis but inhibit mitochondrial fatty acid β-oxidation and export of triglycerides from the liver. Hepatocyte injury and inflammation caused by a number of factors that may include mitochondrial dysfunction, ATP depletion, oxidative stress and lipid peroxidation lead to increased cytotoxic and proinflammatory cytokines and hepatocellular injury. Sustained liver injury leads to hepatic fibrosis, cirrhosis and possibly liver cancer over time.

REFERENCES

[1] Neuschwander-Tetri B. A., Caldwell S. H. (2003). Nonalcoholic steatohepatitis: summary of an AASLD Single Topic Conference. *Hepatology 37,* 1202-1219.

[2] Brunt E. M., Ramrahkiani S., Cordes B. G., Neuschwander-Tetri B. A., Janney C. G., Bacon B. R., Di Bisceglie A. M. (2003). Concurrence of histologic features of steatohepatitis with other forms of chronic liver disease. *Mod. Pathol. 16,* 49-56.

[3] Nomura H., Kashiwagi S., Hayashi J., Kajiyama W., Tani S., Goto M. (1988). Prevalence of fatty liver in a general population of Okinawa, Japan. *Jpn J Med 27,* 142-149.

[4] Bellentani S., Tiribelli C., Saccoccio G., Sodde M., Fratti N., De Martin C., Cristianini G. (1994). Prevalence of chronic liver disease in the general population of northern Italy: the Dionysos Study. *Hepatology 20,* 1442-1449.

[5] Prati D., Taioli E., Zanella A., Della Torre E., Butelli S., Del Vecchio E., Vianello L., Zanuso F., Mozzi F., Milani S., Conte D., Colombo M., Sirchia G. (2002). Updated definitions of healthy ranges for serum alanine aminotransferase levels. *Ann. Intern. Med. 137,* 1-9.

[6] Kim W. R., Brown R. S., Jr., Terrault N. A., El-Serag H. (2002). Burden of liver disease in the United States: summary of a workshop. *Hepatology 36,* 227-242.

[7] McGlynn K. A., London W. T. (2005). Epidemiology and natural history of hepatocellular carcinoma. *Baillieres Best Pract Res Clin Gastroenterol 19,* 3-23.

[8] Browning J. D., Szczepaniak L. S., Dobbins R., Nuremberg P., Horton J. D., Cohen J. C., Grundy S. M., Hobbs H. H. (2004). Prevalence of hepatic

steatosis in an urban population in the United States: impact of ethnicity. *Hepatology 40*, 1387-1395.

[9] Matteoni C. A., Younossi Z. M., Gramlich T., Boparai N., Liu Y. C., McCullough A. J. (1999). Nonalcoholic fatty liver disease: a spectrum of clinical and pathological severity. *Gastroenterology 116*, 1413-1419.

[10] Caldwell S. H., Oelsner D. H., Iezzoni J. C., Hespenheide E. E., Battle E. H., Driscoll C. J. (1999). Cryptogenic cirrhosis: clinical characterization and risk factors for underlying disease. *Hepatology 29*, 664-669.

[11] Poonawala A., Nair S. P., Thuluvath P. J. (2000). Prevalence of obesity and diabetes in patients with cryptogenic cirrhosis: a case-control study. *Hepatology 32*, 689-692.

[12] Ong J., Younossi Z. M., Reddy V., Price L. L., Gramlich T., Mayes J., Boparai N. (2001). Cryptogenic cirrhosis and posttransplantation nonalcoholic fatty liver disease. *Liver Transpl 7*, 797-801.

[13] Charlton M., Kasparova P., Weston S., Lindor K., Maor-Kendler Y., Wiesner R. H., Rosen C. B., Batts K. P. (2001). Frequency of nonalcoholic steatohepatitis as a cause of advanced liver disease. *Liver Transpl 7*, 608-614.

[14] Ratziu V., Bonyhay L., Di Martino V., Charlotte F., Cavallaro L., Sayegh-Tainturier M.-H., Giral P., Grimaldi A., Opolon P., Poynard T. (2002). Survival, liver failure, and hepatocellular carcinoma in obesity-related cryptogenic cirrhosis. *Hepatology 35*, 1485-1493.

[15] Bugianesi E., Leone N., Vanni E., Marchesini G., Brunello F., Carucci P., Musso A., De Paolis P., Capussotti L., Salizzoni M., Rizzetto M. (2002). Expanding the natural history of nonalcoholic steatohepatitis: from cryptogenic cirrhosis to hepatocellular carcinoma. *Gastroenterology 123*, 134-140.

[16] El-Serag H. B. (2004). Hepatocellular carcinoma: recent trends in the United States. *Gastroenterology 127*, S27-34.

[17] Adams L. A., Sanderson S., Lindor K. D., Angulo P. (2005). The histological course of nonalcoholic fatty liver disease: a longitudinal study of 103 patients with sequential liver biopsies. *J. Hepatol. 42*, 132-138.

[18] Marchesini G., Brizi M., Morselli-Labate A. M., Bianchi G., Bugianesi E., McCullough A. J., Forlani G., Melchionda N. (1999). Association of nonalcoholic fatty liver disease with insulin resistance. *Am. J. Med. 107*, 450-455.

[19] Marchesini G., Brizi M., Bianchi G., Tomassetti S., Bugianesi E., Lenzi M., McCullough A. J., Natale S., Forlani G., Melchionda N. (2001).

Nonalcoholic fatty liver disease: a feature of the metabolic syndrome. *Diabetes 50*, 1844-1850.
[20] Chitturi S., Farrell G. C. (2001). Etiopathogenesis of nonalcoholic steatohepatitis. *Sem. Liver Dis. 21*, 27-41.
[21] Sanyal A. J., Campbell-Sargent C., Mirshani F., Rizzo W. B., Contos M. J., Sterling R. K., Luketic V. A., Shiffman M. L., Clore J. (2001). Nonalcoholic steatohepatitis: association of insulin resistance and mitochondrial abnormalities. *Gastroenterology 120*, 1183-1192.
[22] Chitturi S., Abeygunasekera S., Farrell G. C., Holmes-Walker J., Hui J. M., Fung C., Karim R., Lin R., Samarasinghe D., Liddle C., Weltman M., George J. (2002). NASH and insulin resistance: Insulin hypersecretion and specific association with the insulin resistance syndrome. *Hepatology 35*, 373-379.
[23] Seppälä-Lindroos A., Vehkavaara S., Häkkinen A.-M., Goto T., Westerbacka J., Sovijärvi A., Halavaara J., Yki-Järvinen H. (2002). Fat accumulation in the liver is associated with defects in insulin suppression of glucose production and serum free fatty acids independent of obesity in normal men. *J. Clin. Endo. Metab. 87*, 3023-3028.
[24] Pagano G., Pacini G., Musso G., Gambino R., Mecca F., Depetris N., Cassader M., David E., Cavallo-Perin P., Rizzetto M. (2002). Nonalcoholic steatohepatitis, insulin resistance, and metabolic syndrome: further evidence for an etiologic association. *Hepatology 35*, 367-372.
[25] Marchesini G., Bugianesi E., Forlani G., Cerrelli F., Lenzi M., Manini R., Natale S., Vanni E., Melchionda N., Rizzetto M. (2003). Nonalcoholic fatty liver, steatohepatitis, and the metabolic syndrome. *Hepatology 37*, 917-923.
[26] Bugianesi E., Manzini P., D'Antico S., Vanni E., Longo F., Leone N., Massarenti P., Piga A., Marchesini G., Rizzetto M. (2004). Relative contribution of iron burden, HFE mutations, and insulin resistance to fibrosis in nonalcoholic fatty liver. *Hepatology 39*, 179-187.
[27] Reaven G. (2004). The metabolic syndrome or the insulin resistance syndrome? Different names, different concepts, and different goals. *Endocrinol. Metab. Clin. North Am. 33*, 283-303.
[28] Spiegelman B. M., Flier J. S. (2001). Obesity and the regulation of energy balance. *Cell 104*, 531-543.
[29] Minokoshi Y., Kahn C. R., Kahn B. B. (2003). Tissue-specific ablation of the GLUT4 glucose transporter or the insulin receptor challenges assumptions about insulin action and glucose homeostasis. *J. Biol. Chem. 278*, 33609-33612.

[30] Eckel R. H., Grundy S. M., Zimmet P. Z. (2005). The metabolic syndrome. *Lancet 365*, 1415-1428.
[31] Arner P. (2003). The adipocyte in insulin resistance: key molecules and the impact of the thiazolidinediones. *Trends Endocrinol Metab 14*, 137-145.
[32] Le Marchand-Brustel Y., Gual P., Grémeaux T., Gonzalez T., Barrès R., Tanti J.-F. (2003). Fatty acid-induced insulin resistance: role of insulin receptor substrate 1 serine phosphorylation in the retroregulation of insulin signalling. *Biochem. Soc. Trans. 31*, 1152-1156.
[33] Okamoto H., Accili D. (2003). In vivo mutagenesis of the insulin receptor. *J. Biol. Chem. 278*, 28359-28362.
[34] Anai M., Funaki M., Ogihara T., Terasaki J., Inukai K., Katagiri H., Fukushima Y., Yazaki Y., Kikuchi M., Oka Y., Asano T. (1998). Altered expression levels and impaired steps in the pathway to phosphatidylinositol 3-kinase activation via insulin receptor substrates 1 and 2 in Zucker fatty rats. *Diabetes 47*, 13-23.
[35] Taniguchi C. M., Ueki K., Kahn R. (2005). Complementary roles of IRS-1 and IRS-2 in the hepatic regulation of metabolism. *J. Clin. Invest. 115*, 718-727.
[36] Buettner R., Straub R. H., Ottinger I., Woenckhaus M., Scholmerich J., Bollheimer L. C. (2005). Efficient analysis of hepatic glucose output and insulin action using a liver slice culture system. *Horm. Metab. Res. 37*, 127-132.
[37] Fisher S. J., Kahn C. R. (2003). Insulin signaling is required for insulin's direct and indirect action on hepatic glucose production. *J. Clin. Invest. 111*, 463-468.
[38] Jensen M. D., Caruso M., Heiling V., Miles J. M. (1989). Insulin regulation of lipolysis in nondiabetic and IDDM subjects. *Diabetes 38*, 1595-1601.
[39] Smith U., Axelsen M., Carvalho E., Eliasson B., Jansson P. A., Wesslau C. (1999). Insulin signaling and action in fat cells: associations with insulin resistance and type 2 diabetes. *Ann. NY Acad. Sci. 892*, 119-126.
[40] Kahn B. B., Flier J. S. (2000). Obesity and insulin resistance. *J. Clin. Invest. 106*, 473-481.
[41] Summers S. A., Whiteman E. L., Birnbaum M. J. (2000). Insulin signaling in the adipocyte. *Int J Obes 24*, S67-70.
[42] Formiguera X., Cantón A. (2004). Obesity: epidemiology and clinical aspects. *Baillieres Best Pract Res Clin Gastroenterol 18*, 1125-1146.
[43] Pittas A. G., Joseph N. A., Greenberg A. S. (2004). Adipocytokines and insulin resistance. *J. Clin. Endo. Metab. 89*, 447-452.

[44] Bradbury M. W., Berk P. D. (2004). Lipid metabolism in hepatic steatosis. *Clin Liv Dis 8*, 639-671.

[45] Yuan M., Konstantopoulos N., Lee J., Hansen L., Li Z. W., Karin M., Shoelson S. E. (2001). Reversal of obesity- and diet-induced insulin resistance with salicylates or targeted disruption of Ikkβ. *Science 293*, 1673-1677.

[46] Hirosumi J., Tuncman G., Chang L., Görgün C. Z., Uysal K. T., Maeda K., Karin M., Hotamisligil G. S. (2002). A central role of JNK in obesity and insulin resistance. *Nature 420*, 333-336.

[47] Hotamisligil G. S., Peraldi P., Budavari A., Ellis R., White M. F., Spiegelman B. M. (1996). IRS-1-mediated inhibition of insulin receptor tyrosine kinase activity in TNF-α- and obesity-induced insulin resistance. *Science 271*, 665-668.

[48] Peraldi P., Hotamisligil G. S., Buurman W. A., White M. F., Spiegelman B. M. (1996). Tumor necrosis factor (TNF)-α inhibits insulin signaling through stimulation of the p55 TNF receptor and activation of sphingomyelinase. *J. Biol. Chem. 271*, 13018-13022.

[49] Hotamisligil G. S. (1999). The role of TNFα and TNF receptors in obesity and insulin resistance. *J. Int. Med. 245*, 621-625.

[50] Kanety H., Feinstein R., Papa M. Z., Hemi R., Karasik A. (1995). Tumor necrosis factor alpha-induced phosphorylation of insulin receptor substrate-1 (IRS-1). Possible mechanism for suppression of insulin-stimulated tyrosine phosphorylation of IRS-1. *J. Biol. Chem. 270*, 23780-23784.

[51] Paz K., Hemi R., LeRoith D., Karasik A., Elhanany E., Kanety H., Zick Y. (1997). A molecular basis for insulin resistance. Elevated serine/threonine phosphorylation of IRS-1 and IRS-2 inhibits their binding to the juxtamembrane region of the insulin receptor and impairs their ability to undergo insulin-induced tyrosine phosphorylation. *J. Biol. Chem. 272*, 29911-29918.

[52] Sethi J. K., Hotamisligil G. S. (1999). The role of TNF alpha in adipocyte metabolism. *Semin Cell Dev Biol 10*, 19-29.

[53] Kim Y.-B., Shulman G. I., Kahn B. B. (2002). Fatty acid infusion selectively impairs insulin action on Akt1 and protein kinase C lambda /zeta but not on glycogen synthase kinase-3. *J. Biol. Chem. 277*, 32915-32922.

[54] Lam T. K. T., Yoshii H., Haber C. A., Bogdanovic E., Lam L., Fantus I. G., Giacca A. (2002). Free fatty acid-induced hepatic insulin resistance: a potential role for protein kinase C-delta. *Am. J. Physiol. 283*, E682-691.

[55] Samuel V. T., Liu Z.-X., Qu X., Elder B. D., Bilz S., Befroy D., Romanelli A. J., Shulman G. I. (2004). Mechanism of hepatic insulin resistance in nonalcoholic fatty liver disease. *J. Biol. Chem. 279,* 32345-32353.

[56] Yu Y.-H., Zhang Y., Oelkers P., Sturley S. L., Rader D. J., Ginsberg H. N. (2002). Posttranscriptional control of the expression and function of diacylglycerol acyltransferase-1 in mouse adipocytes. *J. Biol. Chem. 277,* 50876-50884.

[57] Chavez J. A., Knotts T. A., Wang L.-P., Li G., Dobrowsky R. T., Florant G. L., Summers S. A. (2003). A role for ceramide, but not diacylglycerol, in the antagonism of insulin signal transduction by saturated fatty acids. *J. Biol. Chem. 278,* 10297-10303.

[58] Kelley D. E., He J., Menshikova E. V., Ritov V. B. (2002). Dysfunction of mitochondria in human skeletal muscle in type 2 diabetes. *Diabetes 51,* 2944-2950.

[59] Shepherd P. R., Kahn B. B. (1999). Glucose transporters and insulin action. Implications for insulin resistance and diabetes mellitus. *N. Engl. J. Med. 341,* 248-257.

[60] Diehl A. M. (2004). Tumor necrosis factor and its potential role in insulin resistance and nonalcoholic fatty liver disease. *Clin Liv Dis 8,* 619-638.

[61] Wellen K. E., Hotamisligil G. S. (2005). Inflammation, stress, and diabetes. *J. Clin. Invest. 115,* 1111-1119.

[62] Yin M. J., Yamamoto Y., Gaynor R. B. (1998). The anti-inflammatory agents aspirin and salicylate inhibit the activity of IκB kinase-β. *Nature 396,* 77-80.

[63] Kim J. K., Kim Y.-J., Fillmore J. J., Chen Y., Moore I., Lee J., Yuan M., Li Z. W., Karin M., Perret P., Shoelson S. E., Shulman G. I. (2001). Prevention of fat-induced insulin resistance by salicylate. *J. Clin. Invest. 108,* 437-446.

[64] Shoelson S. E., Lee J., Yuan M. (2003). Inflammation and the IKK β/IκB/NF-κB axis in obesity- and diet-induced insulin resistance. *International Journal of Obesity & Related Metabolic Disorders: Journal of the International Association for the Study of Obesity 27 Suppl 3,* S49-52.

[65] Hundal R. S., Petersen K. F., Mayerson A. B., Randhawa P. S., Inzucchi S., Shoelson S. E., Shulman G. I. (2002). Mechanism by which high-dose aspirin improves glucose metabolism in type 2 diabetes. *J. Clin. Invest. 109,* 1321-1326.

[66] Cai D., Yuan M., Frantz D. F., Melendez P. A., Hansen L., Lee J., Shoelson S. E. (2005). Local and systemic insulin resistance resulting from hepatic activation of IKK-β and NF-κB. *Nat. Med. 11,* 183-190.

[67] Leclercq I. A., Farrell G. C., Sempoux C., dela Pena A., Horsmans Y. (2004). Curcumin inhibits NF-κB activation and reduces the severity of experimental steatohepatitis in mice. *J. Hepatol. 41*, 926-934.

[68] Perreault M., Marette A. (2001). Targeted disruption of inducible nitric oxide synthase protects against obesity-linked insulin resistance in muscle. *Nat. Med. 7*, 1138-1143.

[69] Emanuelli B., Peraldi P., Filloux C., Chavey C., Freidinger K., Hilton D. J., Hotamisligil G. S., Van Obberghen E. (2001). SOCS-3 inhibits insulin signaling and is up-regulated in response to tumor necrosis factor-α in the adipose tissue of obese mice. *J. Biol. Chem. 276*, 47944-47949.

[70] Ueki K., Kondo T., Tseng Y.-H., Kahn C. R. (2004). Central role of suppressors of cytokine signaling proteins in hepatic steatosis, insulin resistance, and the metabolic syndrome in the mouse. *Proc. Natl. Acad. Sci. 101*, 10422-10427.

[71] Rui L., Yuan M., Frantz D., Shoelson S., White M. F. (2002). SOCS-1 and SOCS-3 block insulin signaling by ubiquitin-mediated degradation of IRS1 and IRS2. *J. Biol. Chem. 277*, 42394-42398.

[72] Johnston J. A., O'Shea J. J. (2003). Matching SOCS with function. *Nat Immunol 4*, 507-509.

[73] Farrell G. C. (2005). Signalling links in the liver: Knitting SOCS with fat and inflammation. *J. Hepatol. 43*, 193-196.

[74] Mori H., Hanada R., Hanada T., Aki D., Mashima R., Nishinakamura H., Torisu T., Chien K. R., Yasukawa H., Yoshimura A. (2004). Socs3 deficiency in the brain elevates leptin sensitivity and confers resistance to diet-induced obesity. *Nat. Med. 10*, 739-743.

[75] Horton J. D., Goldstein J. L., Brown M. S. (2002). SREBPs: activators of the complete program of cholesterol and fatty acid synthesis in the liver. *J. Clin. Invest. 109*, 1125-1131.

[76] Weisberg S. P., McCann D., Desai M., Rosenbaum M., Leibel R. L., Ferrante A. W., Jr. (2003). Obesity is associated with macrophage accumulation in adipose tissue. *J. Clin. Invest. 112*, 1796-1808.

[77] Rockey D. C., Shah V. (2004). Nitric oxide biology and the liver: report of an AASLD research workshop. *Hepatology 39*, 250-257.

[78] Wan G., Ohnomi S., Kato N. (2000). Increased hepatic activity of inducible nitric oxide synthase in rats fed on a high-fat diet. *Biosci Biotechnol Biochem 64*, 555-561.

[79] García-Monzón C., Martín-Pérez E., Iacono O. L., Fernández-Bermejo M., Majano P. L., Apolinario A., Larrañaga E., Moreno-Otero R. (2000).

Characterization of pathogenic and prognostic factors of nonalcoholic steatohepatitis associated with obesity. *J. Hepatol. 33*, 716-724.

[80] Chen Y., Hozawa S., Sawamura S., Sato S., Fukuyama N., Tsuji C., Mine T., Okada Y., Tanino R., Ogushi Y., Nakazawa H. (2005). Deficiency of inducible nitric oxide synthase exacerbates hepatic fibrosis in mice fed high-fat diet. *Biochem. Biophys. Res. Commun. 326*, 45-51.

[81] Donnelly K. L., Smith C. I., Schwarzenberg S. J., Jessurun J., Boldt M. D., Parks E. J. (2005). Sources of fatty acids stored in liver and secreted via lipoproteins in patients with nonalcoholic fatty liver disease. *J. Clin. Invest. 115*, 1343-1351.

[82] Lewis G. F., Steiner G. (1996). Acute effects of insulin in the control of VLDL production in humans. Implications for the insulin-resistant state. *Diabetes Care 19*, 390-393.

[83] Lewis G. F., Uffelman K. D., Szeto L. W., Weller B., Steiner G. (1995). Interaction between free fatty acids and insulin in the acute control of very low density lipoprotein production in humans. *J. Clin. Invest. 95*, 158-166.

[84] Chen Y. D., Golay A., Swislocki A. L., Reaven G. M. (1987). Resistance to insulin suppression of plasma free fatty acid concentrations and insulin stimulation of glucose uptake in noninsulin-dependent diabetes mellitus. *J. Clin. Endo. Metab. 64*, 17-21.

[85] Tamura S., Shimomura I. (2005). Contribution of adipose tissue and de novo lipogenesis to nonalcoholic fatty liver disease. *J. Clin. Invest. 115*, 1139-1142.

[86] Diraison F., Moulin P., Beylot M. (2003). Contribution of hepatic de novo lipogenesis and reesterification of plasma non esterified fatty acids to plasma triglyceride synthesis during non-alcoholic fatty liver disease. *Diabetes Metab. 29*, 478-485.

[87] Hudgins L. C., Hellerstein M. K., Seidman C. E., Neese R. A., Tremaroli J. D., Hirsch J. (2000). Relationship between carbohydrate-induced hypertriglyceridemia and fatty acid synthesis in lean and obese subjects. *J. Lipid Res. 41*, 595-604.

[88] Parks E. J. (2002). Dietary carbohydrate's effects on lipogenesis and the relationship of lipogenesis to blood insulin and glucose concentrations. *Br. J. Nutr. 87 Suppl 2*, S247-253.

[89] Schwarz J.-M., Linfoot P., Dare D., Aghajanian K. (2003). Hepatic de novo lipogenesis in normoinsulinemic and hyperinsulinemic subjects consuming high-fat, low-carbohydrate and low-fat, high-carbohydrate isoenergetic diets. *Am. J. Clin. Nutr. 77*, 43-50.

[90] Araya J., Rodrigo R., Videla L. A., Thielemann L., Orellana M., Pettinelli P., Poniachik J. (2004). Increase in long-chain polyunsaturated fatty acid n - 6/n - 3 ratio in relation to hepatic steatosis in patients with non-alcoholic fatty liver disease. *Clin. Sci. 106,* 635-643.

[91] Shimomura I., Hammer R. E., Richardson J. A., Ikemoto S., Bashmakov Y., Goldstein J. L., Brown M. S. (1998). Insulin resistance and diabetes mellitus in transgenic mice expressing nuclear SREBP-1c in adipose tissue: model for congenital generalized lipodystrophy. *Genes Dev 12,* 3182-3194.

[92] Listenberger L. L., Han X., Lewis S. E., Cases S., Farese R. V., Jr., Ory D. S., Schaffer J. E. (2003). Triglyceride accumulation protects against fatty acid-induced lipotoxicity. *Proc. Natl. Acad. Sci. 100,* 3077-3082.

[93] Kim S. P., Ellmerer M., Van Citters G. W., Bergman R. N. (2003). Primacy of hepatic insulin resistance in the development of the metabolic syndrome induced by an isocaloric moderate-fat diet in the dog. *Diabetes 52,* 2453-2460.

[94] Koo S. H., Dutcher A. K., Towle H. C. (2001). Glucose and insulin function through two distinct transcription factors to stimulate expression of lipogenic enzyme genes in liver. *J. Biol. Chem. 276,* 9437-9445.

[95] Shimomura I., Shimano H., Horton J. D., Goldstein J. L., Brown M. S. (1997). Differential expression of exons 1a and 1c in mRNAs for sterol regulatory element binding protein-1 in human and mouse organs and cultured cells. *J. Clin. Invest. 99,* 838-845.

[96] Brown M. S., Goldstein J. L. (1997). The SREBP pathway: regulation of cholesterol metabolism by proteolysis of a membrane-bound transcription factor. *Cell 89,* 331-340.

[97] Browning J. D., Horton J. D. (2004). Molecular mediators of hepatic steatosis and liver injury. *J. Clin. Invest. 114,* 147-152.

[98] Yahagi N., Shimano H., Hasty A. H., Matsuzaka T., Ide T., Yoshikawa T., Amemiya-Kudo M., Tomita S., Okazaki H., Tamura Y., Iizuka Y., Ohashi K., Osuga J., Harada K., Gotoda T., Nagai R., Ishibashi S., Yamada N. (2002). Absence of sterol regulatory element-binding protein-1 (SREBP-1) ameliorates fatty livers but not obesity or insulin resistance in Lep(ob)/Lep(ob) mice. *J. Biol. Chem. 277,* 19353-19357.

[99] Pai J. T., Guryev O., Brown M. S., Goldstein J. L. (1998). Differential stimulation of cholesterol and unsaturated fatty acid biosynthesis in cells expressing individual nuclear sterol regulatory element-binding proteins. *J. Biol. Chem. 273,* 26138-26148.

[100] Yamashita H., Takenoshita M., Sakurai M., Bruick R. K., Henzel W. J., Shillinglaw W., Arnot D., Uyeda K. (2001). A glucose-responsive

transcription factor that regulates carbohydrate metabolism in the liver. *Proc. Natl. Acad. Sci. 98*, 9116-9121.

[101] Iizuka K., Bruick R. K., Liang G., Horton J. D., Uyeda K. (2004). Deficiency of carbohydrate response element-binding protein (ChREBP) reduces lipogenesis as well as glycolysis. *Proc. Natl. Acad. Sci. 101*, 7281-7286.

[102] Nanji A. A., French S. W. (1989). Dietary linoleic acid is required for development of experimentally induced alcoholic liver injury. *Life Sci. 44*, 223-227.

[103] Nanji A. A., Mendenhall C. L., French S. W. (1989). Beef fat prevents alcoholic liver disease in the rat. *Alcoholism: Clin. Exp. Res. 13*, 15-19.

[104] Ji J., Zhang L., Wang P., Mu Y.-M., Zhu X.-Y., Wu Y.-Y., Yu H., Zhang B., Chen S.-M., Sun X.-Z. (2005). Saturated free fatty acid, palmitic acid, induces apoptosis in fetal hepatocytes in culture. *Exp Toxicol Pathol 56*, 369-376.

[105] Andersen T., Gluud C., Franzmann M.-B., Christoffersen P. (1991). Hepatic effects of dietary weight loss in morbidly obese subjects. *J. Hepatol. 12*, 224-229.

[106] Solga S., Alkhuraishe A. R., Clark J. M., Torbenson M., Greenwald A., Diehl A. M., Magnuson T. (2004). Dietary composition and nonalcoholic fatty liver disease. *Dig. Dis. Sci. 49*, 1578-1583.

[107] Nehra V., Angulo P., Buchman A. L., Lindor K. D. (2001). Nutritional and metabolic considerations in the etiology of nonalcoholic steatohepatitis. *Dig. Dis. Sci. 46*, 2347-2352.

[108] Lonardo A., Loria P. (2002). Apolipoprotein synthesis in nonalcoholic steatohepatitis. *Hepatology 36*, 514-515; discussion 515.

[109] Charlton M., Sreekumar R., Rasmussen D., Lindor K., Nair K. S. (2002). Apolipoprotein synthesis in nonalcoholic steatohepatitis. *Hepatology 35*, 898-904.

[110] Fisher E. A., Ginsberg H. N. (2002). Complexity in the secretory pathway: the assembly and secretion of apolipoprotein B-containing lipoproteins. *J. Biol. Chem. 277*, 17377-17380.

[111] Pan M., Cederbaum A. I., Zhang Y.-L., Ginsberg H. N., Williams K. J., Fisher E. A. (2004). Lipid peroxidation and oxidant stress regulate hepatic apolipoprotein B degradation and VLDL production. *J. Clin. Invest. 113*, 1277-1287.

[112] Cryer D. R., Matsushima T., Marsh J. B., Yudkoff M., Coates P. M., Cortner J. A. (1986). Direct measurement of apolipoprotein B synthesis in

human very low density lipoprotein using stable isotopes and mass spectrometry. *J. Lipid Res. 27,* 508-516.
[113] Halliday D., Venkatesan S., Pacy P. (1993). Apolipoprotein metabolism: a stable-isotope approach. *Am. J. Clin. Nutr. 57,* 726S-730S; discussion 730S-731S.
[114] Wetterau J. R., Lin M. C., Jamil H. (1997). Microsomal triglyceride transfer protein. *Biochim. Biophys. Acta 1345,* 136-150.
[115] Marra F. (2004). NASH: are genes blowing the hits? *J. Hepatol. 40,* 853-856.
[116] Fisher E. A., Pan M., Chen X., Wu X., Wang H., Jamil H., Sparks J. D., Williams K. J. (2001). The triple threat to nascent apolipoprotein B. Evidence for multiple, distinct degradative pathways. *J. Biol. Chem. 276,* 27855-27863.
[117] Adeli K., Taghibiglou C., Van Iderstine S. C., Lewis G. F. (2001). Mechanisms of hepatic very low-density lipoprotein overproduction in insulin resistance. *Trends in Cardiovascular Medicine 11,* 170-176.
[118] Pessayre D., Mansouri A., Fromenty B. (2002). Nonalcoholic steatosis and steatohepatitis. V. Mitochondrial dysfunction in steatohepatitis. *Am J Physiol Gastrointest Liver Physiol 282,* G193-199.
[119] Sparks J. D., Sparks C. E. (1994). Insulin regulation of triacylglycerol-rich lipoprotein synthesis and secretion. *Biochim. Biophys. Acta 1215,* 9-32.
[120] Cummings M. H., Watts G. F., Umpleby A. M., Hennessy T. R., Naoumova R., Slavin B. M., Thompson G. R., Sönksen P. H. (1995). Increased hepatic secretion of very-low-density lipoprotein apolipoprotein B-100 in NIDDM. *Diabetologia 38,* 959-967.
[121] Lewis G. F. (1997). Fatty acid regulation of very low density lipoprotein production. *Curr. Opin. Lipidol. 8,* 146-153.
[122] Julius U. (2003). Influence of plasma free fatty acids on lipoprotein synthesis and diabetic dyslipidemia. *Exp. Clin. Endocrinol. Diabetes 111,* 246-250.
[123] Song J. H., Fujimoto K., Miyazawa T. (2000). Polyunsaturated (n-3) fatty acids susceptible to peroxidation are increased in plasma and tissue lipids of rats fed docosahexaenoic acid-containing oils. *J. Nutr. 130,* 3028-3033.
[124] Tarugi P., Lonardo A., Ballarini G., Grisendi A., Pulvirenti M., Bagni A., Calandra S. (1996). Fatty liver in heterozygous hypobetalipoproteinemia caused by a novel truncated form of apolipoprotein B. *Gastroenterology 111,* 1125-1133.
[125] Tarugi P., Lonardo A., Gabelli C., Sala F., Ballarini G., Cortella I., Previato L., Bertolini S., Cordera R., Calandra S. (2001). Phenotypic expression of

familial hypobetalipoproteinemia in three kindreds with mutations of apolipoprotein B gene. *J. Lipid Res. 42*, 1552-1561.

[126] Pessayre D., Fromenty B. (2005). NASH: a mitochondrial disease. *J. Hepatol. 42*, 928-940.

[127] Foschini M. P., Macchia S., Losi L., Dei Tos A. P., Pasquinelli G., Di Tommaso L., Del Duca S., Roncaroli F., Dal Monte P. R. (1998). Identification of mitochondria in liver biopsies. A study by immunohistochemistry, immunogold and Western blot analysis. *Virchows Archiv 433*, 267-273.

[128] Hassanein T. (2004). Mitochondrial dysfunction in liver disease and organ transplantation. *Mitochondrion 4*, 609-620.

[129] Reddy J. K., Hashimoto T. (2001). Peroxisomal β-oxidation and peroxisome proliferator-activated receptor α: an adaptive metabolic system. *Annu. Rev. Nutr. 21*, 193-230.

[130] Song B. J., Matsunaga T., Hardwick J. P., Park S. S., Veech R. L., Yang C. S., Gelboin H. V., Gonzalez F. J. (1987). Stabilization of cytochrome P450j messenger ribonucleic acid in the diabetic rat. *Mol. Endocrinol. 1*, 542-547.

[131] Hong J. Y., Pan J. M., Gonzalez F. J., Gelboin H. V., Yang C. S. (1987). The induction of a specific form of cytochrome P-450 (P-450j) by fasting. *Biochem. Biophys. Res. Commun. 142*, 1077-1083.

[132] Favreau L. V., Malchoff D. M., Mole J. E., Schenkman J. B. (1987). Responses to insulin by two forms of rat hepatic microsomal cytochrome P-450 that undergo major (RLM6) and minor (RLM5b) elevations in diabetes. *J. Biol. Chem. 262*, 14319-14326.

[133] Dong Z. G., Hong J. Y., Ma Q. A., Li D. C., Bullock J., Gonzalez F. J., Park S. S., Gelboin H. V., Yang C. S. (1988). Mechanism of induction of cytochrome P-450ac (P-450j) in chemically induced and spontaneously diabetic rats. *Arch. Biochem. Biophys. 263*, 29-35.

[134] Bellward G. D., Chang T., Rodrigues B., McNeill J. H., Maines S., Ryan D. E., Levin W., Thomas P. E. (1988). Hepatic cytochrome P-450j induction in the spontaneously diabetic BB rat. *Mol. Pharmacol. 33*, 140-143.

[135] Song B. J., Veech R. L., Saenger P. (1990). Cytochrome P450IIE1 is elevated in lymphocytes from poorly controlled insulin-dependent diabetics. *J. Clin. Endo. Metab. 71*, 1036-1040.

[136] Raucy J. L., Lasker J. M., Kraner J. C., Salazar D. E., Lieber C. S., Corcoran G. B. (1991). Induction of cytochrome P450IIE1 in the obese overfed rat. *Mol. Pharmacol. 39*, 275-280.

[137] Yun Y. P., Casazza J. P., Sohn D. H., Veech R. L., Song B. J. (1992). Pretranslational activation of cytochrome P450IIE during ketosis induced by a high fat diet. *Mol. Pharmacol. 41*, 474-479.
[138] Weltman M. D., Farrell G. C., Liddle C. (1996). Increased hepatocyte CYP2E1 expression in a rat nutritional model of hepatic steatosis with inflammation. *Gastroenterology 111*, 1645-1653.
[139] Weltman M. D., Farrell G. C., Hall P., Ingelman-Sundberg M., Liddle C. (1998). Hepatic cytochrome P450 2E1 is increased in patients with nonalcoholic steatohepatitis. *Hepatology 27*, 128-133.
[140] Enriquez A., Leclercq I., Farrell G. C., Robertson G. (1999). Altered expression of hepatic CYP2E1 and CYP4A in obese, diabetic ob/ob mice, and fa/fa Zucker rats. *Biochem. Biophys. Res. Commun. 255*, 300-306.
[141] Leclercq I. A., Farrell G. C., Field J., Bell D. R., Gonzalez F. J., Robertson G. R. (2000). CYP2E1 and CYP4A as microsomal catalysts of lipid peroxides in murine nonalcoholic steatohepatitis. *J. Clin. Invest. 105*, 1067-1075.
[142] Chalasani N., Gorski J. C., Asghar M. S., Asghar A., Foresman B., Hall S. D., Crabb D. W. (2003). Hepatic cytochrome P450 2E1 activity in nondiabetic patients with nonalcoholic steatohepatitis. *Hepatology 37*, 544-550.
[143] Emery M. G., Fisher J. M., Chien J. Y., Kharasch E. D., Dellinger E. P., Kowdley K. V., Thummel K. E. (2003). CYP2E1 activity before and after weight loss in morbidly obese subjects with nonalcoholic fatty liver disease. *Hepatology 38*, 428-435.
[144] Lieber C. S., Leo M. A., Mak K. M., Xu Y., Cao Q., Ren C., Ponomarenko A., DeCarli L. M. (2004). Model of nonalcoholic steatohepatitis. *Am. J. Clin. Nutr. 79*, 502-509.
[145] Deng Q.-G., She H., Cheng J. H., French S. W., Koop D. R., Xiong S., Tsukamoto H. (2005). Steatohepatitis induced by intragastric overfeeding in mice. *Hepatology 42*, 905-914.
[146] Robertson G., Leclercq I., Farrell G. C. (2001). Nonalcoholic steatosis and steatohepatitis. II. Cytochrome *P*-450 enzymes and oxidative stress. *Am. J. Physiol. 281*, G1135-1139.
[147] Gorsky L. D., Koop D. R., Coon M. J. (1984). On the stoichiometry of the oxidase and monooxygenase reactions catalyzed by liver microsomal cytochrome P-450. Products of oxygen reduction. *J. Biol. Chem. 259*, 6812-6817.
[148] Ekstrom G., Ingelman-Sundberg M. (1989). Rat liver microsomal NADPH-supported oxidase activity and lipid peroxidation dependent on ethanol-

inducible cytochrome P-450 (P-450IIE1). *Biochem. Pharmacol. 38,* 1313-1319.

[149] Yu S., Rao S., Reddy J. K. (2003). Peroxisome proliferator-activated receptors, fatty acid oxidation, steatohepatitis and hepatocarcinogenesis. *Curr Mol Med 3,* 561-572.

[150] Hotamisligil G. S., Shargill N. S., Spiegelman B. M. (1993). Adipose expression of tumor necrosis factor alpha: direct role in obesity-linked insulin resistance. *Science 259,* 87-91.

[151] Hotamisligil G. S. (2003). Inflammation, tumor necrosis factor-□, and insulin resistance. In: LeRoith D., Taylor S. I., Olefsky J., (Eds.), *Diabetes Mellitus: A Fundamental and Clinical Text.* (3rd ed, pp. 953-962). Philadelphia: Lippincott Williams and Wilkins.

[152] Hotamisligil G. S., Spiegelman B. M. (1994). Tumor necrosis factor alpha: a key component of the obesity-diabetes link. *Diabetes 43,* 1271-1278.

[153] Xu H., Barnes G. T., Yang Q., Tan G., Yang D., Chou C. J., Sole J., Nichols A., Ross J. S., Tartaglia L. A., Chen H. (2003). Chronic inflammation in fat plays a crucial role in the development of obesity-related insulin resistance. *J. Clin. Invest. 112,* 1821-1830.

[154] Uysal K. T., Wiesbrock S. M., Marino M. W., Hotamisligil G. S. (1997). Protection from obesity-induced insulin resistance in mice lacking TNF-□ function. *Nature 389,* 610-614.

[155] Kapur S., Bedard S., Marcotte B., Cote C. H., Marette A. (1997). Expression of nitric oxide synthase in skeletal muscle: a novel role for nitric oxide as a modulator of insulin action. *Diabetes 46,* 1691-1700.

[156] Youd J. M., Rattigan S., Clark M. G. (2000). Acute impairment of insulin-mediated capillary recruitment and glucose uptake in rat skeletal muscle in vivo by TNF-□. *Diabetes 49,* 1904-1909.

[157] Furukawa S., Fujita T., Shimabukuro M., Iwaki M., Yamada Y., Nakajima Y., Nakayama O., Makishima M., Matsuda M., Shimomura I. (2004). Increased oxidative stress in obesity and its impact on metabolic syndrome. *J. Clin. Invest. 114,* 1752-1761.

[158] Loria P., Lonardo A., Leonardi F., Fontana C., Carulli L., Verrone A. M., Borsatti A., Bertolotti M., Cassani F., Bagni A., Muratori P., Ganazzi D., Bianchi F. B., Carulli N. (2003). Non-organ-specific autoantibodies in nonalcoholic fatty liver disease: prevalence and correlates. *Dig. Dis. Sci. 48,* 2173-2181.

[159] Park S. H., Kim B. I., Yun J. W., Kim J. W., Park D. I., Cho Y. K., Sung I. K., Park C. Y., Sohn C. I., Jeon W. K., Kim H., Rhee E. J., Lee W. Y., Kim S. W. (2004). Insulin resistance and C-reactive protein as independent risk

factors for non-alcoholic fatty liver disease in non-obese Asian men. *J. Gastroenterol. Hepatol. 19*, 694-698.

[160] Kerner A., Avizohar O., Sella R., Bartha P., Zinder O., Markiewicz W., Levy Y., Brook G. J., Aronson D. (2005). Association between elevated liver enzymes and C-reactive protein: possible hepatic contribution to systemic inflammation in the metabolic syndrome. *Arterioscler. Thromb. Vasc. Biol. 25*, 193-197.

[161] Albano E., Mottaran E., Vidali M., Reale E., Saksena S., Occhino G., Burt A. D., Day C. P. (2005). Immune response towards lipid peroxidation products as a predictor of progression of non-alcoholic fatty liver disease to advanced fibrosis. *Gut 54*, 987-993.

[162] Caldwell S. H., Chang C. Y., Nakamoto R. K., Krugner-Higby L. (2004). Mitochondria in nonalcoholic fatty liver disease. *Clin Liv Dis 8*, 595-617.

[163] Yang S. Q., Lin H. Z., Lane M. D., Clemens M., Diehl A. M. (1997). Obesity increases sensitivity to endotoxin liver injury: implications for the pathogenesis of steatohepatitis. *Proc. Natl. Acad. Sci. 94*, 2557-2562.

[164] Yang S., Zhu H., Li Y., Lin H., Gabrielson K., Trush M. A., Diehl A. M. (2000). Mitochondrial adaptations to obesity-related oxidant stress. *Arch. Biochem. Biophys. 378*, 259-268.

[165] Day C. P., James O. F. (1998). Steatohepatitis: a tale of two "hits"? *Gastroenterology 114*, 842-845.

[166] Yang S., Lin H., Diehl A. M. (2001). Fatty liver vulnerability to endotoxin-induced damage despite NF-κB induction and inhibited caspase 3 activation. *Am J Physiol Gastrointest Liver Physiol 281*, G382-392.

[167] Crespo J., Cayón A., Fernández-Gil P., Hernández-Guerra M., Mayorga M., Domínguez-Díez A., Fernández-Escalante J. C., Pons-Romero F. (2001). Gene expression of tumor necrosis factor α and TNF-receptors, p55 and p75, in nonalcoholic steatohepatitis patients. *Hepatology 34*, 1158-1163.

[168] Chitturi S., Farrell G., Frost L., Kriketos A., Lin R., Fung C., Liddle C., Samarasinghe D., George J. (2002). Serum leptin in NASH correlates with hepatic steatosis but not fibrosis: a manifestation of lipotoxicity? *Hepatology 36*, 403-409.

[169] Maeda N., Shimomura I., Kishida K., Nishizawa H., Matsuda M., Nagaretani H., Furuyama N., Kondo H., Takahashi M., Arita Y., Komuro R., Ouchi N., Kihara S., Tochino Y., Okutomi K., Horie M., Takeda S., Aoyama T., Funahashi T., Matsuzawa Y. (2002). Diet-induced insulin resistance in mice lacking adiponectin/ACRP30. *Nat. Med. 8*, 731-737.

[170] Xu A., Wang Y., Keshaw H., Xu L. Y., Lam K. S., Cooper G. J. (2003). The fat-derived hormone adiponectin alleviates alcoholic and nonalcoholic fatty liver diseases in mice. *J. Clin. Invest. 112*, 91-100.

[171] Hui J. M., Hodge A., Farrell G. C., Kench J. G., Kriketos A., George J. (2004). Beyond insulin resistance in NASH: TNF-α or adiponectin? *Hepatology 40*, 46-54.

[172] Bugianesi E., McCullough A. J., Marchesini G. (2005). Insulin resistance: a metabolic pathway to chronic liver disease. *Hepatology 42*, 987-1000.

[173] Koteish A., Diehl A. M. (2001). Animal models of steatosis. *Sem. Liver Dis. 21*, 89-104.

[174] Oben J. A., Roskams T., Yang S., Lin H., Sinelli N., Li Z., Torbenson M., Thomas S. A., Diehl A. M. (2003). Norepinephrine induces hepatic fibrogenesis in leptin deficient ob/ob mice. *Biochem. Biophys. Res. Commun. 308*, 284-292.

[175] Diehl A. M., Li Z. P., Lin H. Z., Yang S. Q. (2005). Cytokines and the pathogenesis of non-alcoholic steatohepatitis. *Gut 54*, 303-306.

[176] Lord G. M., Matarese G., Howard J. K., Baker R. J., Bloom S. R., Lechler R. I. (1998). Leptin modulates the T-cell immune response and reverses starvation-induced immunosuppression. *Nature 394*, 897-901.

[177] Watson A. M., Poloyac S. M., Howard G., Blouin R. A. (1999). Effect of leptin on cytochrome P-450, conjugation, and antioxidant enzymes in the ob/ob mouse. *Drug Metab Dispos 27*, 695-700.

[178] Leclercq I. A., Field J., Enriquez A., Farrell G. C., Robertson G. R. (2000). Constitutive and inducible expression of hepatic CYP2E1 in leptin-deficient ob/ob mice. *Biochem. Biophys. Res. Commun. 268*, 337-344.

[179] Rinella M. E., Green R. M. (2004). The methionine-choline deficient dietary model of steatohepatitis does not exhibit insulin resistance. *J. Hepatol. 40*, 47-51.

[180] Kashireddy P. V., Rao M. S. (2004). Lack of peroxisome proliferator-activated receptor a in mice enhances methionine and choline deficient diet-induced steatohepatitis. *Hepatology Research 30*, 104-110.

[181] Hashimoto T., Cook W. S., Qi C., Yeldandi A. V., Reddy J. K., Rao M. S. (2000). Defect in peroxisome proliferator-activated receptor alpha-inducible fatty acid oxidation determines the severity of hepatic steatosis in response to fasting. *J. Biol. Chem. 275*, 28918-28928.

[182] Xu Z., Chen L., Leung L., Yen T. S. B., Lee C., Chan J. Y. (2005). Liver-specific inactivation of the Nrf1 gene in adult mouse leads to nonalcoholic steatohepatitis and hepatic neoplasia. *Proc. Natl. Acad. Sci. 102*, 4120-4125.

[183] Day C., Saksena S. (2002). Non-alcoholic steatohepatitis: Definitions and pathogenesis. *J Gastroenterol Hepatol 17 Suppl 3,* S377-S384.

[184] Seki S., Kitada T., Yamada T., Sakaguchi H., Nakatani K., Wakasa K. (2002). In situ detection of lipid peroxidation and oxidative DNA damage in non-alcoholic fatty liver diseases. *J. Hepatol. 37,* 56-62.

[185] Farrell G. C. (2003). Non-alcoholic steatohepatitis: what is it, and why is it important in the Asia-Pacific region? *J. Gastroenterol. Hepatol. 18,* 124-138.

[186] Stärkel P., Sempoux C., Leclercq I., Herin M., Deby C., Desager J.-P., Horsmans Y. (2003). Oxidative stress, KLF6 and transforming growth factor-□ up-regulation differentiate non-alcoholic steatohepatitis progressing to fibrosis from uncomplicated steatosis in rats. *J. Hepatol. 39,* 538-546.

[187] Seki S., Kitada T., Sakaguchi H. (2005). Clinicopathological significance of oxidative cellular damage in non-alcoholic fatty liver diseases. *Hepatology Research 33,* 132-134.

[188] Lavine J. E. (2000). Vitamin E treatment of nonalcoholic steatohepatitis in children: a pilot study. *J. Pediatr. 136,* 734-738.

[189] Hasegawa T., Yoneda M., Nakamura K., Makino I., Terano A. (2001). Plasma transforming growth factor-β1 level and efficacy of □-tocopherol in patients with non-alcoholic steatohepatitis: a pilot study. *Aliment. Pharmacol. Ther. 15,* 1667-1672.

[190] Harrison S. A., Torgerson S., Hayashi P., Ward J., Schenker S. (2003). Vitamin E and vitamin C treatment improves fibrosis in patients with nonalcoholic steatohepatitis. *Am. J. Gastro. 98,* 2485-2490.

[191] Roskams T., Yang S. Q., Koteish A., Durnez A., DeVos R., Huang X., Achten R., Verslype C., Diehl A. M. (2003). Oxidative stress and oval cell accumulation in mice and humans with alcoholic and nonalcoholic fatty liver disease. *Am. J. Pathol. 163,* 1301-1311.

[192] Wallace D. C., Brown M. D., Lott M. T. (1999). Mitochondrial DNA variation in human evolution and disease. *Gene 238,* 211-230.

[193] Lieber C. S. (2004). CYP2E1: from ASH to NASH. *Hepatology Research 28,* 1-11.

[194] Gonzalez F. J. (2005). Role of cytochromes P450 in chemical toxicity and oxidative stress: studies with CYP2E1. *Mutat Res 569,* 101-110.

[195] Lucas D., Farez C., Bardou L. G., Vaisse J., Attali J. R., Valensi P. (1998). Cytochrome P450 2E1 activity in diabetic and obese patients as assessed by chlorzoxazone hydroxylation. *Fundam Clin Pharmacol 12,* 553-558.

[196] Wang Z., Hall S. D., Maya J. F., Li L., Asghar A., Gorski J. C. (2003). Diabetes mellitus increases the in vivo activity of cytochrome P450 2E1 in humans. *Br J Clin Pharmacol 55*, 77-85.

[197] Casazza J. P., Felver M. E., Veech R. L. (1984). The metabolism of acetone in rat. *J. Biol. Chem. 259*, 231-236.

[198] Koop D. R., Tierney D. J. (1990). Multiple mechanisms in the regulation of ethanol-inducible cytochrome P450IIE1. *Bioessays 12*, 429-435.

[199] Woodcroft K. J., Hafner M. S., Novak R. F. (2002). Insulin signaling in the transcriptional and posttranscriptional regulation of CYP2E1 expression. *Hepatology 35*, 263-273.

[200] Woodcroft K. J., Novak R. F. (1997). Insulin effects on CYP2E1, 2B, 3A, and 4A expression in primary cultured rat hepatocytes. *Chem. Biol. Interact. 107*, 75-91.

[201] Woodcroft K. J., Novak R. F. (1999). Insulin differentially affects xenobiotic-enhanced, cytochrome P-450 (CYP)2E1, CYP2B, CYP3A, and CYP4A expression in primary cultured rat hepatocytes. *J. Pharmacol. Exp. Therap. 289*, 1121-1127.

[202] De Waziers I., Garlatti M., Bouguet J., Beaune P. H., Barouki R. (1995). Insulin down-regulates cytochrome P450 2B and 2E expression at the post-transcriptional level in the rat hepatoma cell line. *Mol. Pharmacol. 47*, 474-479.

[203] Leclercq I., Horsmans Y., Desager J. P., Pauwels S., Geubel A. P. (1999). Dietary restriction of energy and sugar results in a reduction in human cytochrome P450 2E1 activity. *Br. J. Nutr. 82*, 257-262.

[204] Nieto N., Friedman S. L., Greenwel P., Cederbaum A. I. (1999). CYP2E1-mediated oxidative stress induces collagen type I expression in rat hepatic stellate cells. *Hepatology 30*, 987-996.

[205] Casini A., Pellegrini G., Ceni E., Salzano R., Parola M., Robino G., Milani S., Dianzani M. U., Surrenti C. (1998). Human hepatic stellate cells express class I alcohol dehydrogenase and aldehyde dehydrogenase but not cytochrome P4502E1. *J. Hepatol. 28*, 40-45.

[206] George D. K., Goldwurm S., MacDonald G. A., Cowley L. L., Walker N. I., Ward P. J., Jazwinska E. C., Powell L. W. (1998). Increased hepatic iron in nonalcoholic steatohepatitis is associated with increased fibrosis. *Gastroenterology 114*, 311-318.

[207] Bonkovsky H. L., Jawaid Q., Tortorelli K., LeClair P., Cobb J., Lambrecht R. W., Banner B. F. (1999). Non-alcoholic steatohepatitis and iron: increased prevalence of mutations of the HFE gene in non-alcoholic steatohepatitis. *J. Hepatol. 31*, 421-429.

[208] Younossi Z. M., Gramlich T., Bacon B. R., Matteoni C. A., Boparai N., O'Neill R., McCullough A. J. (1999). Hepatic iron and nonalcoholic fatty liver disease. *Hepatology 30,* 847-850.

[209] Chitturi S., Weltman M., Farrell G. C., McDonald D., Kench J., Liddle C., Samarasinghe D., Lin R., Abeygunasekera S., George J. (2002). HFE mutations, hepatic iron, and fibrosis: ethnic-specific association of NASH with C282Y but not with fibrotic severity. *Hepatology 36,* 142-149.

[210] Ruhl C. E., Everhart J. E. (2003). Relation of elevated serum alanine aminotransferase activity with iron and antioxidant levels in the United States. *Gastroenterology 124,* 1821-1829.

[211] Facchini F. S., Hua N. W., Stoohs R. A. (2002). Effect of iron depletion in carbohydrate-intolerant patients with clinical evidence of nonalcoholic fatty liver disease. *Gastroenterology 122,* 931-939.

[212] Cortez-Pinto H., Chatham J., Chacko V. P., Arnold C., Rashid A., Diehl A. M. (1999). Alterations in liver ATP homeostasis in human nonalcoholic steatohepatitis: a pilot study. *J. Am. Med. Assoc. 282,* 1659-1664.

[213] Caldwell S. H., Swerdlow R. H., Khan E. M., Iezzoni J. C., Hespenheide E. E., Parks J. K., Parker W. D., Jr. (1999). Mitochondrial abnormalities in non-alcoholic steatohepatitis. *J. Hepatol. 31,* 430-434.

[214] Le T. H., Caldwell S. H., Redick J. A., Sheppard B. L., Davis C. A., Arseneau K. O., Iezzoni J. C., Hespenheide E. E., Al-Osaimi A., Peterson T. C. (2004). The zonal distribution of megamitochondria with crystalline inclusions in nonalcoholic steatohepatitis. *Hepatology 39,* 1423-1429.

[215] Caldwell S. H., Hespenheide E. E., Redick J. A., Iezzoni J. C., Battle E. H., Sheppard B. L. (2001). A pilot study of a thiazolidinedione, troglitazone, in nonalcoholic steatohepatitis. *Am. J. Gastro. 96,* 519-525.

[216] Powell E. E., Cooksley W. G., Hanson R., Searle J., Halliday J. W., Powell L. W. (1990). The natural history of nonalcoholic steatohepatitis: a follow-up study of forty-two patients for up to 21 years. *Hepatology 11,* 74-80.

[217] Pérez-Carreras M., Del Hoyo P., Martín M. A., Rubio J. C., Martín A., Castellano G., Colina F., Arenas J., Solis-Herruzo J. A. (2003). Defective hepatic mitochondrial respiratory chain in patients with nonalcoholic steatohepatitis. *Hepatology 38,* 999-1007.

[218] Ibdah J. A., Perlegas P., Zhao Y., Angdisen J., Borgerink H., Shadoan M. K., Wagner J. D., Matern D., Rinaldo P., Cline J. M. (2005). Mice heterozygous for a defect in mitochondrial trifunctional protein develop hepatic steatosis and insulin resistance. *Gastroenterology 128,* 1381-1390.

[219] Feldstein A. E., Werneburg N. W., Canbay A., Guicciardi M. E., Bronk S. F., Rydzewski R., Burgart L. J., Gores G. J. (2004). Free fatty acids promote

hepatic lipotoxicity by stimulating TNF-α expression via a lysosomal pathway. *Hepatology 40,* 185-194.

[220] Chavin K. D., Yang S., Lin H. Z., Chatham J., Chacko V. P., Hoek J. B., Walajtys-Rode E., Rashid A., Chen C. H., Huang C. C., Wu T. C., Lane M. D., Diehl A. M. (1999). Obesity induces expression of uncoupling protein-2 in hepatocytes and promotes liver ATP depletion. *J. Biol. Chem. 274,* 5692-5700.

[221] Tsuboyama-Kasaoka N., Takahashi M., Kim H., Ezaki O. (1999). Up-regulation of liver uncoupling protein-2 mRNA by either fish oil feeding or fibrate administration in mice. *Biochem. Biophys. Res. Commun. 257,* 879-885.

[222] Memon R. A., Hotamisligil G. S., Wiesbrock S. M., Uysal K. T., Faggioni R., Moser A. H., Feingold K. R., Grunfeld C. (2000). Upregulation of uncoupling protein 2 mRNA in genetic obesity: lack of an essential role for leptin, hyperphagia, increased tissue lipid content, and TNF-α. *Biochim. Biophys. Acta 1484,* 41-50.

[223] Baffy G., Zhang C.-Y., Glickman J. N., Lowell B. B. (2002). Obesity-related fatty liver is unchanged in mice deficient for mitochondrial uncoupling protein 2. *Hepatology 35,* 753-761.

[224] Bowyer B. A., Miles J. M., Haymond M. W., Fleming C. R. (1988). L-carnitine therapy in home parenteral nutrition patients with abnormal liver tests and low plasma carnitine concentrations. *Gastroenterology 94,* 434-438.

[225] Harper P., Wadström C., Backman L., Cederblad G. (1995). Increased liver carnitine content in obese women. *Am. J. Clin. Nutr. 61,* 18-25.

[226] Moller D. E. (2001). New drug targets for type 2 diabetes and the metabolic syndrome. *Nature 414,* 821-827.

[227] Perseghin G., Petersen K., Shulman G. I. (2003). Cellular mechanism of insulin resistance: potential links with inflammation. *International Journal of Obesity & Related Metabolic Disorders: Journal of the International Association for the Study of Obesity 27 Suppl 3,* S6-11.

[228] Lee Y., Hirose H., Ohneda M., Johnson J. H., McGarry J. D., Unger R. H. (1994). Beta-cell lipotoxicity in the pathogenesis of non-insulin-dependent diabetes mellitus of obese rats: impairment in adipocyte-beta-cell relationships. *Proc. Natl. Acad. Sci. 91,* 10878-10882.

[229] Unger R. H. (2002). Lipotoxic diseases. *Annu. Rev. Med. 53,* 319-336.

[230] Unger R. H., Orci L. (2002). Lipoapoptosis: its mechanism and its diseases. *Biochim. Biophys. Acta 1585,* 202-212.

[231] Yaney G. C., Corkey B. E. (2003). Fatty acid metabolism and insulin secretion in pancreatic beta cells. *Diabetologia 46*, 1297-1312.

[232] Boucher A., Lu D., Burgess S. C., Telemaque-Potts S., Jensen M. V., Mulder H., Wang M.-Y., Unger R. H., Sherry A. D., Newgard C. B. (2004). Biochemical mechanism of lipid-induced impairment of glucose-stimulated insulin secretion and reversal with a malate analogue. *J. Biol. Chem. 279*, 27263-27271.

[233] Joseph J. W., Koshkin V., Saleh M. C., Sivitz W. I., Zhang C.-Y., Lowell B. B., Chan C. B., Wheeler M. B. (2004). Free fatty acid-induced beta-cell defects are dependent on uncoupling protein 2 expression. *J. Biol. Chem. 279*, 51049-51056.

[234] Heller R. A., Kronke M. (1994). Tumor necrosis factor receptor-mediated signaling pathways. *J. Cell Biol. 126*, 5-9.

[235] Mayeux P. R. (1997). Pathobiology of lipopolysaccharide. *J Toxicol Environ Health 51*, 415-435.

[236] Wang X. (2001). The expanding role of mitochondria in apoptosis. *Genes Dev 15*, 2922-2933.

[237] Heyninck K., Beyaert R. (2001). Crosstalk between NF-κB-activating and apoptosis-inducing proteins of the TNF-receptor complex. *Mol Cell Biol Res Commun 4*, 259-265.

[238] Guicciardi M. E., Gores G. J. (2005). Apoptosis: a mechanism of acute and chronic liver injury. *Gut 54*, 1024-1033.

[239] Van Antwerp D. J., Martin S. J., Kafri T., Green D. R., Verma I. M. (1996). Suppression of TNF-α-induced apoptosis by NF-κB. *Science 274*, 787-789.

[240] Hockenbery D., Nunez G., Milliman C., Schreiber R. D., Korsmeyer S. J. (1990). Bcl-2 is an inner mitochondrial membrane protein that blocks programmed cell death. *Nature 348*, 334-336.

[241] Takehara T., Liu X., Fujimoto J., Friedman S. L., Takahashi H. (2001). Expression and role of Bcl-xL in human hepatocellular carcinomas. *Hepatology 34*, 55-61.

[242] Maedler K., Oberholzer J., Bucher P., Spinas G. A., Donath M. Y. (2003). Monounsaturated fatty acids prevent the deleterious effects of palmitate and high glucose on human pancreatic beta-cell turnover and function. *Diabetes 52*, 726-733.

[243] Schaffer J. E. (2003). Lipotoxicity: when tissues overeat. *Curr. Opin. Lipidol. 14*, 281-287.

[244] Yost R. L., Duerson M. C., Russell W. L., O'Leary J. P. (1979). Doxycycline in the prevention of hepatic dysfunction: an evaluation of its use following jejunoileal bypass in humans. *Arch. Surg. 114*, 931-934.

[245] Drenick E. J., Fisler J., Johnson D. (1982). Hepatic steatosis after intestinal bypass--prevention and reversal by metronidazole, irrespective of protein-calorie malnutrition. *Gastroenterology 82*, 535-548.

[246] Enomoto N., Yamashina S., Kono H., Schemmer P., Rivera C. A., Enomoto A., Nishiura T., Nishimura T., Brenner D. A., Thurman R. G. (1999). Development of a new, simple rat model of early alcohol-induced liver injury based on sensitization of Kupffer cells. *Hepatology 29*, 1680-1689.

[247] Pappo I., Becovier H., Berry E. M., Freund H. R. (1991). Polymyxin B reduces cecal flora, TNF production and hepatic steatosis during total parenteral nutrition in the rat. *J. Surg. Res. 51*, 106-112.

[248] Nazim M., Stamp G., Hodgson H. J. (1989). Non-alcoholic steatohepatitis associated with small intestinal diverticulosis and bacterial overgrowth. *Hepato-Gastroenterol 36*, 349-351.

[249] Solga S. F., Diehl A. M. (2003). Non-alcoholic fatty liver disease: lumen-liver interactions and possible role for probiotics. *J. Hepatol. 38*, 681-687.

[250] Nair S., Cope K., Risby T. H., Diehl A. M. (2001). Obesity and female gender increase breath ethanol concentration: potential implications for the pathogenesis of nonalcoholic steatohepatitis. *Am. J. Gastro. 96*, 1200-1204.

[251] Wigg A. J., Roberts-Thomson I. C., Dymock R. B., McCarthy P. J., Grose R. H., Cummins A. G. (2001). The role of small intestinal bacterial overgrowth, intestinal permeability, endotoxaemia, and tumour necrosis factor □ in the pathogenesis of non-alcoholic steatohepatitis. *Gut 48*, 206-211.

[252] Pappo I., Bercovier H., Berry E., Gallilly R., Feigin E., Freund H. R. (1995). Antitumor necrosis factor antibodies reduce hepatic steatosis during total parenteral nutrition and bowel rest in the rat. *J. Paren. Ent. Nutr. 19*, 80-82.

[253] Loguercio C., De Simone T., Federico A., Terracciano F., Tuccillo C., Di Chicco M., Carteni M. (2002). Gut-liver axis: a new point of attack to treat chronic liver damage? *Am. J. Gastro. 97*, 2144-2146.

[254] Li Z., Yang S., Lin H., Huang J., Watkins P. A., Moser A. B., DeSimone C., Song X., Diehl A. M. (2003). Probiotics and antibodies to TNF inhibit inflammatory activity and improve nonalcoholic fatty liver disease. *Hepatology 37*, 343-350.

[255] Rosen E. D., Spiegelman B. M. (2000). Molecular regulation of adipogenesis. *Annu Rev Cell Dev Biol 16*, 145-171.

[256] Hotamisligil G. S. (2003). Inflammatory pathways and insulin action. *International Journal of Obesity & Related Metabolic Disorders: Journal of the International Association for the Study of Obesity 27 Suppl 3*, S53-55.

[257] Havel P. J. (2004). Update on adipocyte hormones: regulation of energy balance and carbohydrate/lipid metabolism. *Diabetes 53 Suppl 1*, S143-151.
[258] Rajala M. W., Scherer P. E. (2003). Minireview: The adipocyte--at the crossroads of energy homeostasis, inflammation, and atherosclerosis. *Endocrinology 144*, 3765-3773.
[259] Pond C. M. (2005). Adipose tissue and the immune system. *Prostaglandins Leukot Essent Fatty Acids 73*, 17-30.
[260] Fujioka S., Matsuzawa Y., Tokunaga K., Tarui S. (1987). Contribution of intra-abdominal fat accumulation to the impairment of glucose and lipid metabolism in human obesity. *Metab. Clin. Exp. 36*, 54-59.
[261] Rendell M., Hulthen U. L., Tornquist C., Groop L., Mattiasson I. (2001). Relationship between abdominal fat compartments and glucose and lipid metabolism in early postmenopausal women. *J. Clin. Endo. Metab. 86*, 744-749.
[262] Cnop M., Landchild M. J., Vidal J., Havel P. J., Knowles N. G., Carr D. R., Wang F., Hull R. L., Boyko E. J., Retzlaff B. M., Walden C. E., Knopp R. H., Kahn S. E. (2002). The concurrent accumulation of intra-abdominal and subcutaneous fat explains the association between insulin resistance and plasma leptin concentrations : distinct metabolic effects of two fat compartments. *Diabetes 51*, 1005-1015.
[263] Wajchenberg B. L., Giannella-Neto D., da Silva M. E., Santos R. F. (2002). Depot-specific hormonal characteristics of subcutaneous and visceral adipose tissue and their relation to the metabolic syndrome. *Horm. Metab. Res. 34*, 616-621.
[264] Misra A., Vikram N. K. (2003). Clinical and pathophysiological consequences of abdominal adiposity and abdominal adipose tissue depots. *Nutrition 19*, 457-466.
[265] Klein S., Fontana L., Young V. L., Coggan A. R., Kilo C., Patterson B. W., Mohammed B. S. (2004). Absence of an effect of liposuction on insulin action and risk factors for coronary heart disease. *N. Engl. J. Med. 350*, 2549-2557.
[266] Considine R. V., Sinha M. K., Heiman M. L., Kriauciunas A., Stephens T. W., Nyce M. R., Ohannesian J. P., Marco C. C., McKee L. J., Bauer T. L., et al. (1996). Serum immunoreactive-leptin concentrations in normal-weight and obese humans. *N. Engl. J. Med. 334*, 292-295.
[267] Ahima R., Osei S. Y. (2004). Leptin and appetite control in lipodystrophy. *J. Clin. Endo. Metab. 89*, 4254-4257.

[268] Potter J. J., Womack L., Mezey E., Anania F. A. (1998). Transdifferentiation of rat hepatic stellate cells results in leptin expression. *Biochem. Biophys. Res. Commun. 244*, 178-182.

[269] Ikejima K., Okumura K., Lang T., Honda H., Abe W., Yamashina S., Enomoto N., Takei Y., Sato N. (2005). The role of leptin in progression of non-alcoholic fatty liver disease. *Hepatology Research 33*, 151-154.

[270] Zhang Y., Proenca R., Maffei M., Barone M., Leopold L., Friedman J. M. (1994). Positional cloning of the mouse obese gene and its human homologue. *Nature 372*, 425-432.

[271] Tartaglia L. A., Dembski M., Weng X., Deng N., Culpepper J., Devos R., Richards G. J., Campfield L. A., Clark F. T., Deeds J., Muir C., Sanker S., Moriarty A., Moore K. J., Smutko J. S., Mays G. G., Wool E. A., Monroe C. A., Tepper R. I. (1995). Identification and expression cloning of a leptin receptor, OB-R. *Cell 83*, 1263-1271.

[272] Vaisse C., Halaas J. L., Horvath C. M., Darnell J. E., Jr., Stoffel M., Friedman J. M. (1996). Leptin activation of Stat3 in the hypothalamus of wild-type and ob/ob mice but not db/db mice. *Nat. Genet. 14*, 95-97.

[273] Wang Y., Kuropatwinski K. K., White D. W., Hawley T. S., Hawley R. G., Tartaglia L. A., Baumann H. (1997). Leptin receptor action in hepatic cells. *J. Biol. Chem. 272*, 16216-16223.

[274] Saxena N. K., Ikeda K., Rockey D. C., Friedman S. L., Anania F. A. (2002). Leptin in hepatic fibrosis: evidence for increased collagen production in stellate cells and lean littermates of ob/ob mice. *Hepatology 35*, 762-771.

[275] Giannini E., Botta F., Cataldi A., Tenconi G. L., Ceppa P., Barreca T., Testa R. (1999). Leptin levels in nonalcoholic steatohepatitis and chronic hepatitis C. *Hepato-Gastroenterol 46*, 2422-2425.

[276] Ikejima K., Takei Y., Honda H., Hirose M., Yoshikawa M., Zhang Y. J., Lang T., Fukuda T., Yamashina S., Kitamura T., Sato N. (2002). Leptin receptor-mediated signaling regulates hepatic fibrogenesis and remodeling of extracellular matrix in the rat. *Gastroenterology 122*, 1399-1410.

[277] Leclercq I. A., Farrell G. C., Schriemer R., Robertson G. R. (2002). Leptin is essential for the hepatic fibrogenic response to chronic liver injury. *J. Hepatol. 37*, 206-213.

[278] Nakao K., Nakata K., Ohtsubo N., Maeda M., Moriuchi T., Ichikawa T., Hamasaki K., Kato Y., Eguchi K., Yukawa K., Ishii N. (2002). Association between nonalcoholic fatty liver, markers of obesity, and serum leptin level in young adults. *Am. J. Gastro. 97*, 1796-1801.

[279] Chalasani N., Crabb D. W., Cummings O. W., Kwo P. Y., Asghar A., Pandya P. K., Considine R. V. (2003). Does leptin play a role in the

pathogenesis of human nonalcoholic steatohepatitis? *Am. J. Gastro. 98*, 2771-2776.
[280] Angulo P., Alba L. M., Petrovic L. M., Adams L. A., Lindor K. D., Jensen M. D. (2004). Leptin, insulin resistance, and liver fibrosis in human nonalcoholic fatty liver disease. *J. Hepatol. 41*, 943-949.
[281] Campfield L. A., Smith F. J., Guisez Y., Devos R., Burn P. (1995). Recombinant mouse OB protein: evidence for a peripheral signal linking adiposity and central neural networks. *Science 269*, 546-549.
[282] Halaas J. L., Gajiwala K. S., Maffei M., Cohen S. L., Chait B. T., Rabinowitz D., Lallone R. L., Burley S. K., Friedman J. M. (1995). Weight-reducing effects of the plasma protein encoded by the obese gene. *Science 269*, 543-546.
[283] Oral E. A., Simha V., Ruiz E., Andewelt A., Premkumar A., Snell P., Wagner A. J., DePaoli A. M., Reitman M. L., Taylor S. I., Gorden P., Garg A. (2002). Leptin-replacement therapy for lipodystrophy. *N. Engl. J. Med. 346*, 570-578.
[284] Shimomura I., Hammer R. E., Ikemoto S., Brown M. S., Goldstein J. L. (1999). Leptin reverses insulin resistance and diabetes mellitus in mice with congenital lipodystrophy. *Nature 401*, 73-76.
[285] Gavrilova O., Marcus-Samuels B., Graham D., Kim J. K., Shulman G. I., Castle A. L., Vinson C., Eckhaus M., Reitman M. (2000). Surgical implantation of adipose tissue reverses diabetes in lipoatrophic mice. *J. Clin. Invest. 105*, 271-278.
[286] Loffreda S., Yang S. Q., Lin H. Z., Karp C. L., Brengman M. L., Wang D. J., Klein A. S., Bulkley G. B., Bao C., Noble P. W., Lane M. D., Diehl A. M. (1998). Leptin regulates proinflammatory immune responses. *FASEB J. 12*, 57-65.
[287] Lee F. Y., Li Y., Yang E. K., Yang S. Q., Lin H. Z., Trush M. A., Dannenberg A. J., Diehl A. M. (1999). Phenotypic abnormalities in macrophages from leptin-deficient, obese mice. *Am. J. Physiol. 276*, C386-394.
[288] Santos-Alvarez J., Goberna R., Sanchez-Margalet V. (1999). Human leptin stimulates proliferation and activation of human circulating monocytes. *Cell Immunol 194*, 6-11.
[289] Fantuzzi G., Faggioni R. (2000). Leptin in the regulation of immunity, inflammation, and hematopoiesis. *J Leukoc Biol 68*, 437-446.
[290] Faggioni R., Feingold K. R., Grunfeld C. (2001). Leptin regulation of the immune response and the immunodeficiency of malnutrition. *FASEB J. 15*, 2565-2571.

[291] Farooqi I. S., Matarese G., Lord G. M., Keogh J. M., Lawrence E., Agwu C., Sanna V., Jebb S. A., Perna F., Fontana S., Lechler R. I., DePaoli A. M., O'Rahilly S. (2002). Beneficial effects of leptin on obesity, T cell hyporesponsiveness, and neuroendocrine/metabolic dysfunction of human congenital leptin deficiency. *J. Clin. Invest. 110,* 1093-1103.

[292] Lee Y., Wang M. Y., Kakuma T., Wang Z. W., Babcock E., McCorkle K., Higa M., Zhou Y. T., Unger R. H. (2001). Liporegulation in diet-induced obesity. The antisteatotic role of hyperleptinemia. *J. Biol. Chem. 276,* 5629-5635.

[293] Javor E. D., Ghany M. G., Cochran E. K., Oral E. A., DePaoli A. M., Premkumar A., Kleiner D. E., Gorden P. (2005). Leptin reverses nonalcoholic steatohepatitis in patients with severe lipodystrophy. *Hepatology 41,* 753-760.

[294] Montague C. T., Farooqi I. S., Whitehead J. P., Soos M. A., Rau H., Wareham N. J., Sewter C. P., Digby J. E., Mohammed S. N., Hurst J. A., Cheetham C. H., Earley A. R., Barnett A. H., Prins J. B., O'Rahilly S. (1997). Congenital leptin deficiency is associated with severe early-onset obesity in humans. *Nature 387,* 903-908.

[295] Clement K., Vaisse C., Lahlou N., Cabrol S., Pelloux V., Cassuto D., Gourmelen M., Dina C., Chambaz J., Lacorte J. M., Basdevant A., Bougneres P., Lebouc Y., Froguel P., Guy-Grand B. (1998). A mutation in the human leptin receptor gene causes obesity and pituitary dysfunction. *Nature 392,* 398-401.

[296] Friedman J. M., Leibel R. L., Siegel D. S., Walsh J., Bahary N. (1991). Molecular mapping of the mouse ob mutation. *Genomics 11,* 1054-1062.

[297] Campfield L. A., Smith F. J., Burn P. (1996). The OB protein (leptin) pathway--a link between adipose tissue mass and central neural networks. *Horm. Metab. Res. 28,* 619-632.

[298] Mantzoros C. S., Flier J. S. (2000). Editorial: leptin as a therapeutic agent--trials and tribulations. *J. Clin. Endo. Metab. 85,* 4000-4002.

[299] Lebovitz H. E. (2003). The relationship of obesity to the metabolic syndrome. *Int J Clin Pract Supplement.,* 18-27.

[300] Rosenbaum M., Nicolson M., Hirsch J., Murphy E., Chu F., Leibel R. L. (1997). Effects of weight change on plasma leptin concentrations and energy expenditure. *J. Clin. Endo. Metab. 82,* 3647-3654.

[301] Ziccardi P., Nappo F., Giugliano G., Esposito K., Marfella R., Cioffi M., D'Andrea F., Molinari A. M., Giugliano D. (2002). Reduction of inflammatory cytokine concentrations and improvement of endothelial

functions in obese women after weight loss over one year. *Circulation 105,* 804-809.
[302] Yamauchi T., Kamon J., Ito Y., Tsuchida A., Yokomizo T., Kita S., Sugiyama T., Miyagishi M., Hara K., Tsunoda M., Murakami K., Ohteki T., Uchida S., Takekawa S., Waki H., Tsuno N. H., Shibata Y., Terauchi Y., Froguel P., Tobe K., Koyasu S., Taira K., Kitamura T., Shimizu T., Nagai R., Kadowaki T. (2003). Cloning of adiponectin receptors that mediate antidiabetic metabolic effects. *Nature 423,* 762-769.
[303] Matsuzawa Y., Funahashi T., Kihara S., Shimomura I. (2004). Adiponectin and metabolic syndrome. *Arterioscler. Thromb. Vasc. Biol. 24,* 29-33.
[304] Yu Y.-H., Ginsberg H. N. (2005). Adipocyte signaling and lipid homeostasis: sequelae of insulin-resistant adipose tissue. *Circ. Res. 96,* 1042-1052.
[305] Kubota N., Terauchi Y., Yamauchi T., Kubota T., Moroi M., Matsui J., Eto K., Yamashita T., Kamon J., Satoh H., Yano W., Froguel P., Nagai R., Kimura S., Kadowaki T., Noda T. (2002). Disruption of adiponectin causes insulin resistance and neointimal formation. *J. Biol. Chem. 277,* 25863-25866.
[306] Nawrocki A. R., Scherer P. E. (2004). The delicate balance between fat and muscle: adipokines in metabolic disease and musculoskeletal inflammation. *Curr Opin Pharmacol 4,* 281-289.
[307] Bajaj M., Suraamornkul S., Piper P., Hardies L. J., Glass L., Cersosimo E., Pratipanawatr T., Miyazaki Y., DeFronzo R. A. (2004). Decreased plasma adiponectin concentrations are closely related to hepatic fat content and hepatic insulin resistance in pioglitazone-treated type 2 diabetic patients. *J. Clin. Endo. Metab. 89,* 200-206.
[308] Ma K., Cabrero A., Saha P. K., Kojima H., Li L., Chang B. H.-J., Paul A., Chan L. (2002). Increased β-oxidation but no insulin resistance or glucose intolerance in mice lacking adiponectin. *J. Biol. Chem. 277,* 34658-34661.
[309] Kappes A., Loffler G. (2000). Influences of ionomycin, dibutyryl-cycloAMP and tumour necrosis factor-α on intracellular amount and secretion of apM1 in differentiating primary human preadipocytes. *Horm. Metab. Res. 32,* 548-554.
[310] Fasshauer M., Klein J., Neumann S., Eszlinger M., Paschke R. (2002). Hormonal regulation of adiponectin gene expression in 3T3-L1 adipocytes. *Biochem. Biophys. Res. Commun. 290,* 1084-1089.
[311] Bruun J. M., Lihn A. S., Verdich C., Pedersen S. B., Toubro S., Astrup A., Richelsen B. (2003). Regulation of adiponectin by adipose tissue-derived

cytokines: in vivo and in vitro investigations in humans. *Am. J. Physiol. 285*, E527-533.

[312] Berg A. H., Combs T. P., Scherer P. E. (2002). ACRP30/adiponectin: an adipokine regulating glucose and lipid metabolism. *Trends Endocrinol Metab 13*, 84-89.

[313] Yamauchi T., Kamon J., Minokoshi Y., Ito Y., Waki H., Uchida S., Yamashita S., Noda M., Kita S., Ueki K., Eto K., Akanuma Y., Froguel P., Foufelle F., Ferre P., Carling D., Kimura S., Nagai R., Kahn B. B., Kadowaki T. (2002). Adiponectin stimulates glucose utilization and fatty-acid oxidation by activating AMP-activated protein kinase. *Nat. Med. 8*, 1288-1295.

[314] Yokota T., Oritani K., Takahashi I., Ishikawa J., Matsuyama A., Ouchi N., Kihara S., Funahashi T., Tenner A. J., Tomiyama Y., Matsuzawa Y. (2000). Adiponectin, a new member of the family of soluble defense collagens, negatively regulates the growth of myelomonocytic progenitors and the functions of macrophages. *Blood 96*, 1723-1732.

[315] Ouchi N., Kihara S., Arita Y., Nishida M., Matsuyama A., Okamoto Y., Ishigami M., Kuriyama H., Kishida K., Nishizawa H., Hotta K., Muraguchi M., Ohmoto Y., Yamashita S., Funahashi T., Matsuzawa Y. (2001). Adipocyte-derived plasma protein, adiponectin, suppresses lipid accumulation and class A scavenger receptor expression in human monocyte-derived macrophages. *Circulation 103*, 1057-1063.

[316] Arita Y., Kihara S., Ouchi N., Takahashi M., Maeda K., Miyagawa J., Hotta K., Shimomura I., Nakamura T., Miyaoka K., Kuriyama H., Nishida M., Yamashita S., Okubo K., Matsubara K., Muraguchi M., Ohmoto Y., Funahashi T., Matsuzawa Y. (1999). Paradoxical decrease of an adipose-specific protein, adiponectin, in obesity. *Biochem. Biophys. Res. Commun. 257*, 79-83.

[317] Weyer C., Funahashi T., Tanaka S., Hotta K., Matsuzawa Y., Pratley R. E., Tataranni P. A. (2001). Hypoadiponectinemia in obesity and type 2 diabetes: close association with insulin resistance and hyperinsulinemia. *J. Clin. Endo. Metab. 86*, 1930-1935.

[318] Hoffstedt J., Arvidsson E., Sjolin E., Wahlen K., Arner P. (2004). Adipose tissue adiponectin production and adiponectin serum concentration in human obesity and insulin resistance. *J. Clin. Endo. Metab. 89*, 1391-1396.

[319] Lindsay R. S., Funahashi T., Hanson R. L., Matsuzawa Y., Tanaka S., Tataranni P. A., Knowler W. C., Krakoff J. (2002). Adiponectin and development of type 2 diabetes in the Pima Indian population. *Lancet 360*, 57-58.

[320] Vuppalanchi R., Marri S., Kolwankar D., Considine R. V., Chalasani N. (2005). Is adiponectin involved in the pathogenesis of nonalcoholic steatohepatitis? A preliminary human study. *J. Clin. Gastroenterol. 39,* 237-242.

[321] Kaser S., Moschen A., Cayon A., Kaser A., Crespo J., Pons-Romero F., Ebenbichler C. F., Patsch J. R., Tilg H. (2005). Adiponectin and its receptors in non-alcoholic steatohepatitis. *Gut 54,* 117-121.

[322] Hotamisligil G. S., Arner P., Caro J. F., Atkinson R. L., Spiegelman B. M. (1995). Increased adipose tissue expression of tumor necrosis factor-□ in human obesity and insulin resistance. *J. Clin. Invest. 95,* 2409-2415.

[323] Kern P. A., Saghizadeh M., Ong J. M., Bosch R. J., Deem R., Simsolo R. B. (1995). The expression of tumor necrosis factor in human adipose tissue. Regulation by obesity, weight loss, and relationship to lipoprotein lipase. *J. Clin. Invest. 95,* 2111-2119.

[324] Pfeiffer A., Janott J., Mohlig M., Ristow M., Rochlitz H., Busch K., Schatz H., Schifferdecker E. (1997). Circulating tumor necrosis factor alpha is elevated in male but not in female patients with type II diabetes mellitus. *Horm. Metab. Res. 29,* 111-114.

[325] Winkler G., Salamon F., Harmos G., Salamon D., Speer G., Szekeres O., Hajos P., Kovacs M., Simon K., Cseh K. (1998). Elevated serum tumor necrosis factor-□ concentrations and bioactivity in Type 2 diabetics and patients with android type obesity. *Diabetes Res Clin Pract 42,* 169-174.

[326] Katsuki A., Sumida Y., Murashima S., Murata K., Takarada Y., Ito K., Fujii M., Tsuchihashi K., Goto H., Nakatani K., Yano Y. (1998). Serum levels of tumor necrosis factor-α are increased in obese patients with noninsulin-dependent diabetes mellitus. *J. Clin. Endo. Metab. 83,* 859-862.

[327] Dandona P., Weinstock R., Thusu K., Abdel-Rahman E., Aljada A., Wadden T. (1998). Tumor necrosis factor-α in sera of obese patients: fall with weight loss. *J. Clin. Endo. Metab. 83,* 2907-2910.

[328] Paolisso G., Rizzo M. R., Mazziotti G., Tagliamonte M. R., Gambardella A., Rotondi M., Carella C., Giugliano D., Varricchio M., D'Onofrio F. (1998). Advancing age and insulin resistance: role of plasma tumor necrosis factor-α. *Am. J. Physiol. 275,* E294-299.

[329] Lin H. Z., Yang S. Q., Chuckaree C., Kuhajda F., Ronnet G., Diehl A. M. (2000). Metformin reverses fatty liver disease in obese, leptin-deficient mice. *Nat. Med. 6,* 998-1003.

[330] Hu E., Kim J. B., Sarraf P., Spiegelman B. M. (1996). Inhibition of adipogenesis through MAP kinase-mediated phosphorylation of PPARgamma. *Science 274,* 2100-2103.

[331] Xu H., Sethi J. K., Hotamisligil G. S. (1999). Transmembrane tumor necrosis factor (TNF)-α inhibits adipocyte differentiation by selectively activating TNF receptor 1. *J. Biol. Chem. 274*, 26287-26295.

[332] MacDougald O. A., Mandrup S. (2002). Adipogenesis: forces that tip the scales. *Trends Endocrinol Metab 13*, 5-11.

[333] Kern P. A., Ranganathan S., Li C., Wood L., Ranganathan G. (2001). Adipose tissue tumor necrosis factor and interleukin-6 expression in human obesity and insulin resistance. *Am. J. Physiol. 280*, E745-751.

[334] Bastard J. P., Jardel C., Bruckert E., Blondy P., Capeau J., Laville M., Vidal H., Hainque B. (2000). Elevated levels of interleukin 6 are reduced in serum and subcutaneous adipose tissue of obese women after weight loss. *J. Clin. Endo. Metab. 85*, 3338-3342.

[335] Warne J. P. (2003). Tumour necrosis factor alpha: a key regulator of adipose tissue mass. *J. Endocrin. 177*, 351-355.

[336] Marchesini G., Brizi M., Bianchi G., Tomassetti S., Zoli M., Melchionda N. (2001). Metformin in non-alcoholic steatohepatitis (letter). *Lancet 358*, 893-894.

[337] Neuschwander-Tetri B. A., Brunt E. M., Wehmeier K. R., Sponseller C., Hampton K., Bacon B. R. (2003). Interim results of a pilot study demonstrating the early effects of the PPAR-γ ligand rosiglitazone on insulin sensitivity, aminotransferases, hepatic steatosis and body weight in patients with non-alcoholic steatohepatitis. *J. Hepatol. 38*, 434-440.

[338] Neuschwander-Tetri B. A., Brunt E. M., Wehmeier K. R., Oliver D., Bacon B. R. (2003). Improved nonalcoholic steatohepatitis after 48 weeks of treatment with the PPAR-γ ligand rosiglitazone. *Hepatology 38*, 1008-1017.

[339] Promrat K., Lutchman G., Uwaifo G. I., Freedman R. J., Soza A., Heller T., Doo E., Ghany M., Premkumar A., Park Y., Liang T. J., Yanovski J. A., Kleiner D. E., Hoofnagle J. H. (2004). A pilot study of pioglitazone treatment for nonalcoholic steatohepatitis. *Hepatology 39*, 188-196.

[340] Fried S. K., Bunkin D. A., Greenberg A. S. (1998). Omental and subcutaneous adipose tissues of obese subjects release interleukin-6: depot difference and regulation by glucocorticoid. *J. Clin. Endo. Metab. 83*, 847-850.

[341] Fernandez-Real J. M., Vayreda M., Richart C., Gutierrez C., Broch M., Vendrell J., Ricart W. (2001). Circulating interleukin 6 levels, blood pressure, and insulin sensitivity in apparently healthy men and women. *J. Clin. Endo. Metab. 86*, 1154-1159.

[342] Senn J. J., Klover P. J., Nowak I. A., Mooney R. A. (2002). Interleukin-6 induces cellular insulin resistance in hepatocytes. *Diabetes 51*, 3391-3399.

[343] Senn J. J., Klover P. J., Nowak I. A., Zimmers T. A., Koniaris L. G., Furlanetto R. W., Mooney R. A. (2003). Suppressor of cytokine signaling-3 (SOCS-3), a potential mediator of interleukin-6-dependent insulin resistance in hepatocytes. *J. Biol. Chem. 278,* 13740-13746.

[344] Vozarova B., Weyer C., Hanson K., Tataranni P. A., Bogardus C., Pratley R. E. (2001). Circulating interleukin-6 in relation to adiposity, insulin action, and insulin secretion. *Obes. Res. 9,* 414-417.

[345] Bastard J.-P., Maachi M., Van Nhieu J. T., Jardel C., Bruckert E., Grimaldi A., Robert J.-J., Capeau J., Hainque B. (2002). Adipose tissue IL-6 content correlates with resistance to insulin activation of glucose uptake both in vivo and in vitro. *J. Clin. Endo. Metab. 87,* 2084-2089.

[346] Savage D. B., Sewter C. P., Klenk E. S., Segal D. G., Vidal-Puig A., Considine R. V., O'Rahilly S. (2001). Resistin / Fizz3 expression in relation to obesity and peroxisome proliferator-activated receptor-gamma action in humans. *Diabetes 50,* 2199-2202.

[347] Steppan C. M., Lazar M. A. (2004). The current biology of resistin. *J. Int. Med. 255,* 439-447.

[348] Steppan C. M., Bailey S. T., Bhat S., Brown E. J., Banerjee R. R., Wright C. M., Patel H. R., Ahima R. S., Lazar M. A. (2001). The hormone resistin links obesity to diabetes. *Nature 409,* 307-312.

[349] Rajala M. W., Obici S., Scherer P. E., Rossetti L. (2003). Adipose-derived resistin and gut-derived resistin-like molecule-β selectively impair insulin action on glucose production. *J. Clin. Invest. 111,* 225-230.

[350] Guebre-Xabier M., Yang S., Lin H. Z., Schwenk R., Krzych U., Diehl A. M. (2000). Altered hepatic lymphocyte subpopulations in obesity-related murine fatty livers: potential mechanism for sensitization to liver damage. *Hepatology 31,* 633-640.

[351] Li Z., Lin H., Yang S., Diehl A. M. (2002). Murine leptin deficiency alters Kupffer cell production of cytokines that regulate the innate immune system. *Gastroenterology 123,* 1304-1310.

[352] Li Z., Oben J. A., Yang S., Lin H., Stafford E. A., Soloski M. J., Thomas S. A., Diehl A. M. (2004). Norepinephrine regulates hepatic innate immune system in leptin-deficient mice with nonalcoholic steatohepatitis. *Hepatology 40,* 434-441.

[353] Li Z., Soloski M. J., Diehl A. M. (2005). Dietary factors alter hepatic innate immune system in mice with nonalcoholic fatty liver disease. *Hepatology 42,* 880-885.

[354] Jones D. E. J. (2005). Fat is an immuno-regulatory issue. *Hepatology 42,* 755-758.

[355] Feldstein A. E., Canbay A., Angulo P., Taniai M., Burgart L. J., Lindor K. D., Gores G. J. (2003). Hepatocyte apoptosis and fas expression are prominent features of human nonalcoholic steatohepatitis. *Gastroenterology 125*, 437-443.

[356] Feldstein A. E., Canbay A., Guicciardi M. E., Higuchi H., Bronk S. F., Gores G. J. (2003). Diet associated hepatic steatosis sensitizes to Fas mediated liver injury in mice. *J. Hepatol. 39*, 978-983.

[357] Ribeiro P. S., Cortez-Pinto H., Sola S., Castro R. E., Ramalho R. M., Baptista A., Moura M. C., Camilo M. E., Rodrigues C. M. P. (2004). Hepatocyte apoptosis, expression of death receptors, and activation of NF-κB in the liver of nonalcoholic and alcoholic steatohepatitis patients. *Am. J. Gastro. 99*, 1708-1717.

[358] Higuchi M., Aggarwal B. B., Yeh E. T. (1997). Activation of CPP32-like protease in tumor necrosis factor-induced apoptosis is dependent on mitochondrial function. *J. Clin. Invest. 99*, 1751-1758.

[359] Washington K., Wright K., Shyr Y., Hunter E. B., Olson S., Raiford D. S. (2000). Hepatic stellate cell activation in nonalcoholic steatohepatitis and fatty liver. *Hum. Pathol. 31*, 822-828.

[360] Reynaert H., Thompson M. G., Thomas T., Geerts A. (2002). Hepatic stellate cells: role in microcirculation and pathophysiology of portal hypertension. *Gut 50*, 571-581.

[361] Pinzani M., Rombouts K., Colagrande S. (2005). Fibrosis in chronic liver diseases: diagnosis and management. *J. Hepatol. 42 Suppl*, S22-36.

[362] Bataller R., Brenner D. A. (2005). Liver fibrosis.[erratum appears in J Clin Invest. 2005 Apr;115(4):1100]. *Journal of Clinical Investigation 115*, 209-218.

[363] George J., Pera N., Phung N., Leclercq I., Yun Hou J., Farrell G. C. (2003). Lipid peroxidation, stellate cell activation and hepatic fibrogenesis in a rat model of chronic steatohepatitis. *J. Hepatol. 39*, 756-764.

[364] Paradis V., Perlemuter G., Bonvoust F., Dargere D., Parfait B., Vidaud M., Conti M., Huet S., Ba N., Buffet C., Bedossa P. (2001). High glucose and hyperinsulinemia stimulate connective tissue growth factor expression: a potential mechanism involved in progression to fibrosis in nonalcoholic steatohepatitis. *Hepatology 34*, 738-744.

[365] Ratziu V., Giral P., Charlotte F., Bruckert E., Thibault V., Theodorou I., Khalil L., Turpin G., Opolon P., Poynard T. (2000). Liver fibrosis in overweight patients. *Gastroenterology 118*, 1117-1123.

[366] Chojkier M., Houglum K., Solis-Herruzo J., Brenner D. A. (1989). Stimulation of collagen gene expression by ascorbic acid in cultured human fibroblasts. A role for lipid peroxidation? *J. Biol. Chem. 264,* 16957-16962.

[367] Parola M., Pinzani M., Casini A., Albano E., Poli G., Gentilini A., Gentilini P., Dianzani M. U. (1993). Stimulation of lipid peroxidation or 4-hydroxynonenal treatment increases procollagen alpha 1 (I) gene expression in human liver fat-storing cells. *Biochem. Biophys. Res. Commun. 194,* 1044-1050.

[368] Bissell D. M., Roulot D., George J. (2001). Transforming growth factor □ and the liver. *Hepatology 34,* 859-867.

[369] Marra F. (2002). Leptin and liver fibrosis: a matter of fat. *Gastroenterology 122,* 1529-1532.

[370] Honda H., Ikejima K., Hirose M., Yoshikawa J., Lang T., Enomoto N., Kitamura T., Takai Y., Sato N. (2002). Leptin is required for fibrogenic responses induced by thioacetamide in the murine liver. *Hepatology 36,* 12-21.

[371] Potter J. J., Mezey E. (2002). Leptin deficiency reduces but does not eliminate the development of hepatic fibrosis in mice infected with Schistosoma mansoni. *Liver 22,* 173-177.

[372] Saxena N. K., Saliba G., Floyd J. J., Anania F. A. (2003). Leptin induces increased alpha2(I) collagen gene expression in cultured rat hepatic stellate cells. *J. Cell. Biochem. 89,* 311-320.

[373] Yoshiji H., Kuriyama S., Yoshii J., Ikenaka Y., Noguchi R., Nakatani T., Tsujinoue H., Fukui H. (2001). Angiotensin-II type 1 receptor interaction is a major regulator for liver fibrosis development in rats. *Hepatology 34,* 745-750.

[374] Yokohama S., Yoneda M., Haneda M., Okamoto S., Okada M., Aso K., Hasegawa T., Tokusashi Y., Miyokawa N., Nakamura K. (2004). Therapeutic efficacy of an angiotensin II receptor antagonist in patients with nonalcoholic steatohepatitis. *Hepatology 40,* 1222-1225.

[375] Cotrim H. P., Parana R., Braga E., Lyra L. (2000). Nonalcoholic steatohepatitis and hepatocellular carcinoma: natural history? *Am. J. Gastro. 95,* 3018-3019.

[376] Zen Y., Katayanagi K., Tsuneyama K., Harada K., Araki I., Nakanuma Y. (2001). Hepatocellular carcinoma arising in non-alcoholic steatohepatitis. *Pathol. Int. 51,* 127-131.

[377] Orikasa H., Ohyama R., Tsuka N., Eyden B. P., Yamazaki K. (2001). Lipid-rich clear-cell hepatocellular carcinoma arising in non-alcoholic

steatohepatitis in a patient with diabetes mellitus. *J Submicrosc Cytol Pathol 33,* 195-200.

[378] Shimada M., Hashimoto E., Taniai M., Hasegawa K., Okuda H., Hayashi N., Takasaki K., Ludwig J. (2002). Hepatocellular carcinoma in patients with non-alcoholic steatohepatitis. *J. Hepatol. 37,* 154-160.

[379] Yoshioka Y., Hashimoto E., Yatsuji S., Kaneda H., Taniai M., Tokushige K., Shiratori K. (2004). Nonalcoholic steatohepatitis: cirrhosis, hepatocellular carcinoma, and burnt-out NASH. *J Gastroenterol 39,* 1215-1218.

[380] Mori S., Yamasaki T., Sakaida I., Takami T., Sakaguchi E., Kimura T., Kurokawa F., Maeyama S., Okita K. (2004). Hepatocellular carcinoma with nonalcoholic steatohepatitis. *J Gastroenterol 39,* 391-396.

[381] Cuadrado A., Orive A., Garcia-Suarez C., Dominguez A., Fernandez-Escalante J. C., Crespo J., Pons-Romero F. (2005). Non-alcoholic steatohepatitis (NASH) and hepatocellular carcinoma. *Obesity Surgery 15,* 442-446.

[382] Marrero J. A., Fontana R. J., Su G. I., Conjeevaram H. S., Emick D. M., Lok A. S. (2002). NAFLD may be a common underlying liver disease in patients with hepatocellular carcinoma in the United States. *Hepatology 36,* 1349-1354.

[383] Hui J. M., Kench J., Chitturi S., Sud A., Farrell G. C., Byth K., Hall P., Khan M., George D. K. (2003). Long-term outcomes of cirrhosis in nonalcoholic steatohepatitis compared with hepatitis C. *Hepatology 38,* 420-427.

[384] Hashimoto E., Taniai M., Kaneda H., Tokushige K., Hasegawa K., Okuda H., Shiratori K., Takasaki K. (2004). Comparison of hepatocellular carcinoma patients with alcoholic liver disease and nonalcoholic steatohepatitis. *Alcoholism: Clin. Exp. Res. 28,* 164S-168S.

[385] Horie Y., Suzuki A., Kataoka E., Sasaki T., Hamada K., Sasaki J., Mizuno K., Hasegawa G., Kishimoto H., Iizuka M., Naito M., Enomoto K., Watanabe S., Mak T. W., Nakano T. (2004). Hepatocyte-specific Pten deficiency results in steatohepatitis and hepatocellular carcinomas. *J. Clin. Invest. 113,* 1774-1783.

[386] Soga M., Kishimoto Y., Kawamura Y., Inagaki S., Makino S., Saibara T. (2003). Spontaneous development of hepatocellular carcinomas in the FLS mice with hereditary fatty liver. *Cancer Lett. 196,* 43-48.

[387] Jones M. E., Thorburn A. W., Britt K. L., Hewitt K. N., Wreford N. G., Proietto J., Oz O. K., Leury B. J., Robertson K. M., Yao S., Simpson E. R.

(2000). Aromatase-deficient (ArKO) mice have a phenotype of increased adiposity. *Proc. Natl. Acad. Sci. 97*, 12735-12740.

[388] Lombardi B. (1966). Considerations on the pathogenesis of fatty liver. *Lab. Invest. 15*, 1-20.

[389] Hautekeete M. L., Degott C., Benhamou J. P. (1990). Microvesicular steatosis of the liver. *Acta Clin Belg 45*, 311-326.

[390] Bacon B. R., Farahvash M. J., Janney C. G., Neuschwander-Tetri B. A. (1994). Nonalcoholic steatohepatitis: an expanded clinical entity. *Gastroenterology 107*, 1103-1109.

[391] Fraser J. L., Antonioli D. A., Chopra S., Wang H. H. (1995). Prevalence and nonspecificity of microvesicular fatty change in the liver. *Mod. Pathol. 8*, 65-70.

[392] Brunt E. M., Tiniakos D. G. (2002). Pathology of steatohepatitis. *Baillieres Best Pract Res Clin Gastroenterol 16*, 691-707.

[393] Kleiner D. E., Brunt E. M., Van Natta M., Behling C., Contos M. J., Cummings O. W., Ferrell L. D., Liu Y.-C., Torbenson M. S., Unalp-Arida A., Yeh M., McCullough A. J., Sanyal A. J., Nonalcoholic Steatohepatitis Clinical Research N. (2005). Design and validation of a histological scoring system for nonalcoholic fatty liver disease. *Hepatology 41*, 1313-1321.

[394] Pande S. V., Blanchaer M. C. (1971). Reversible inhibition of mitochondrial adenosine diphosphate phosphorylation by long chain acyl coenzyme A esters. *J. Biol. Chem. 246*, 402-411.

[395] Burt A. D., Mutton A., Day C. P. (1998). Diagnosis and interpretation of steatosis and steatohepatitis. *Semin. Diagn. Pathol. 15*, 246-258.

[396] Brunt E. M. (2004). Nonalcoholic steatohepatitis. *Sem. Liver Dis. 24*, 3-20.

[397] Tilg H., Diehl A. M. (2000). Cytokines in alcoholic and nonalcoholic steatohepatitis. *N. Engl. J. Med. 343*, 1467-1476.

[398] Diehl A. M. (2002). Nonalcoholic steatosis and steatohepatitis IV. Nonalcoholic fatty liver disease abnormalities in macrophage function and cytokines. *Am. J. Physiol. 282*, G1-5.

[399] Schwimmer J. B., Behling C., Newbury R., Deutsch R., Nievergelt C., Schork N. J., Lavine J. E. (2005). Histopathology of pediatric nonalcoholic fatty liver disease. *Hepatology 42*, 641-649.

[400] Abraham S., Furth E. E. (1994). Receiver operating characteristic analysis of glycogenated nuclei in liver biopsy specimens: quantitative evaluation of their relationship with diabetes and obesity. *Hum. Pathol. 25*, 1063-1068.

[401] Nagore N., Scheuer P. J. (1988). The pathology of diabetic hepatitis. *J. Pathol. 156*, 155-160.

[402] Gramlich T., Kleiner D. E., McCullough A. J., Matteoni C. A., Boparai N., Younossi Z. M. (2004). Pathologic features associated with fibrosis in nonalcoholic fatty liver disease. *Hum. Pathol. 35*, 196-199.

[403] Denk H., Stumptner C., Zatloukal K. (2000). Mallory bodies revisited. *J. Hepatol. 32*, 689-702.

[404] Dunkelberg J. C., Feranchak A. P., Fitz J. G. (2001). Liver cell volume regulation: size matters. *Hepatology 33*, 1349-1352.

[405] Janig E., Stumptner C., Fuchsbichler A., Denk H., Zatloukal K. (2005). Interaction of stress proteins with misfolded keratins. *Eur. J. Cell. Biol. 84*, 329-339.

[406] Evans C. D. J., Oien K. A., MacSween R. N. M., Mills P. R. (2002). Non-alcoholic steatohepatitis: a common cause of progressive chronic liver injury? *J. Clin. Pathol. 55*, 689-692.

[407] Harrison S. A., Torgerson S., Hayashi P. H. (2003). The natural history of nonalcoholic fatty liver disease: a clinical histopathological study. *Am. J. Gastro. 98*, 2042-2047.

[408] Fassio E., Alvarez E., Dominguez N., Landeira G., Longo C. (2004). Natural history of nonalcoholic steatohepatitis: a longitudinal study of repeat liver biopsies. *Hepatology 40*, 820-826.

[409] Sacks D. B., McDonald J. M. (1996). The pathogenesis of type II diabetes mellitus. A polygenic disease. *Am. J. Clin. Pathol. 105*, 149-156.

[410] Powell E. E., Searle J., Mortimer R. (1989). Steatohepatitis associated with limb lipodystrophy. *Gastroenterology 97*, 1022-1024.

[411] Struben V. M. D., Hespenheide E. E., Caldwell S. (2000). Nonalcoholic steatohepatitis and cryptogenic cirrhosis within kindreds. *Am. J. Med. 108*, 9-13.

[412] Caldwell S. H., Harris D. M., Patrie J. T., Hespenheide E. E. (2002). Is NASH underdiagnosed among African Americans? *Am. J. Gastro. 97*, 1496-1500.

[413] Browning J. D., Kumar K. S., Saboorian M. H., Thiele D. L. (2004). Ethnic differences in the prevalence of cryptogenic cirrhosis. *Am. J. Gastro. 99*, 292-298.

[414] Weston S. R., Leyden W., Murphy R., Bass N. M., Bell B. P., Manos M. M., Terrault N. A. (2005). Racial and ethnic distribution of nonalcoholic fatty liver in persons with newly diagnosed chronic liver disease. *Hepatology 41*, 372-379.

[415] Solga S. F., Clark J. M., Alkhuraishi A. R., Torbenson M., Tabesh A., Schweitzer M., Diehl A. M., Magnuson T. H. (2005). Race and comorbid

factors predict nonalcoholic fatty liver disease histopathology in severely obese patients. *Surgery for Obesity and Related Diseases 1*, 6-11.
[416] Xanthakos S., Khoury P., O'Brien K., Dardzinski B., Donnelly L., Bucuvalas J., Daniels S. (2005). Low prevalence of nonalcoholic fatty liver disease in young adult women despite high prevalence of obesity. *Hepatology 42*, 613A.
[417] Bernard S., Touzet S., Personne I., Lapras V., Bondon P. J., Berthezène F., Moulin P. (2000). Association between microsomal triglyceride transfer protein gene polymorphism and the biological features of liver steatosis in patients with type II diabetes. *Diabetologia 43*, 995-999.
[418] Valenti L., Fracanzani A. L., Dongiovanni P., Santorelli G., Branchi A., Taioli E., Fiorelli G., Fargion S. (2002). Tumor necrosis factor alpha promoter polymorphisms and insulin resistance in nonalcoholic fatty liver disease. *Gastroenterology 122*, 274-280.
[419] Sreekumar R., Rosado B., Rasmussen D., Charlton M. (2003). Hepatic gene expression in histologically progressive nonalcoholic steatohepatitis. *Hepatology 38*, 244-251.
[420] Younossi Z. M., Baranova A., Ziegler K., Del Giacco L., Schlauch K., Born T. L., Elariny H., Gorreta F., Vanmeter A., Younoszai A., Ong J. P., Goodman Z., Chandhoke V. (2005). A genomic and proteomic study of the spectrum of nonalcoholic fatty liver disease. *Hepatology 42*, 665-674.
[421] Day C. P. (2004). The potential role of genes in nonalcoholic fatty liver disease. *Clin Liv Dis 8*, 673-691.
[422] Grundy S. M., Cleeman J. I., Daniels S. R., Donato K. A., Eckel R. H., Franklin B. A., Gordon D. J., Krauss R. M., Savage P. J., Smith S. C., Jr., Spertus J. A., Costa F., American Heart A., National Heart L., Blood I. (2005). Diagnosis and management of the metabolic syndrome: an American Heart Association/National Heart, Lung, and Blood Institute Scientific Statement. *Circulation 112*, 2735-2752.

INDEX

#

4-hydroxynonenal, 25, 30, 93

A

abdominal, 83
abnormalities, viii, 3, 4, 6, 12, 15, 19, 22, 33, 34, 35, 38, 39, 40, 41, 42, 51, 59, 63, 79, 85, 95
acetone, 78
acid, vii, 2, 5, 6, 7, 9, 11, 12, 14, 15, 16, 17, 18, 19, 20, 21, 22, 25, 26, 28, 31, 34, 35, 36, 37, 41, 42, 43, 44, 46, 50, 52, 56, 59, 64, 65, 67, 68, 69, 70, 71, 74, 76, 81, 88, 93
actin, 1, 47
activated receptors, 74
activation, 7, 10, 11, 15, 22, 27, 32, 37, 41, 45, 46, 47, 48, 49, 57, 64, 65, 66, 67, 73, 75, 84, 85, 91, 92
activators, 67
acute, 23, 52, 68, 81
Adams, 62, 85
adaptation, 15
adenoma, 50
adenosine, 95
adipocyte, 14, 22, 44, 64, 65, 80, 83, 90
adipocytes, 4, 5, 6, 7, 20, 39, 40, 41, 42, 43, 44, 59, 66, 87
adipocytokines, vii, viii, 2, 7, 22, 26, 39, 48, 51, 59, 64
adipogenic, 50
adiponectin, 1, 29, 39, 42, 43, 44, 75, 76, 87, 88, 89
adipose, vii, 2, 5, 6, 7, 8, 12, 13, 14, 15, 16, 17, 20, 22, 25, 39, 40, 41, 42, 43, 44, 54, 67, 68, 69, 83, 85, 86, 87, 88, 89, 90
adipose tissue, vii, 2, 5, 6, 7, 8, 12, 13, 14, 15, 17, 20, 22, 25, 39, 40, 41, 42, 43, 44, 54, 67, 68, 69, 83, 85, 86, 87, 89, 90
adiposity, 22, 83, 85, 91, 95
administration, 33, 38, 40, 41, 42, 44, 48, 80
adult, 29, 53, 56, 76, 97
adults, 3, 84
African American, 55, 96
African Americans, 55, 96
age, 18, 23, 32, 38, 48, 49, 50, 89
agent, 86
agents, 23, 43, 66
aggregation, 52, 55
aging, 34, 36
alanine, 33, 61, 79
alanine aminotransferase, 33, 61, 79
albumin, 19
alcohol, v, 3, 17, 49, 56, 78, 82

alcohol abuse, v, 3
alcohol consumption, 3
alcoholic liver disease, 70, 94
aldehydes, 30
alpha, 2, 7, 9, 65, 74, 76, 89, 90, 93, 97
alternative, 21
alters, 91
American Heart Association, 97
amino, 13, 14
amino acid, 13, 14
amino acids, 13, 14
angiotensin, 49, 93
Angiotensin, 49, 93
Angiotensin II, 49, 93
angiotensin II receptor antagonist, 49, 93
animal models, vii, 19, 21, 22, 27, 28, 39, 43, 44, 49
animal studies, 11, 32, 38
animals, 5, 11, 25, 31, 36, 38
anion, 22
antagonism, 39, 66
antagonist, 49, 93
anti-apoptotic, 10, 37
antibiotic, 38
antibiotics, 38
antibody, 23, 43
antidiabetic, 87
anti-inflammatory, 23, 41, 42, 45, 66
anti-inflammatory agents, 23, 66
antioxidant, 10, 19, 29, 30, 35, 50, 56, 76, 79
antioxidants, viii, 10, 25, 30, 31, 56, 57
antitrypsin, 57
apoptosis, 15, 17, 30, 37, 38, 39, 43, 45, 46, 49, 54, 70, 81, 92
apoptotic, 10, 37, 45, 46
apoptotic cells, 45
apoptotic effect, 10, 37
appetite, 83
APS, 1, 5, 9
argument, 25
ascorbic, 93
ascorbic acid, 93
Asia, 77
Asian, 75
aspirin, 10, 66

associations, 64
assumptions, 63
atherosclerosis, 83
ATP, 20, 30, 31, 34, 36, 59, 79, 80
attention, 44
attractiveness, 30
autoantibodies, 23, 74
autocrine, 7, 43, 47
availability, 18

B

bacteria, 38
bacterial, 26, 38, 82
bariatric surgery, 55, 57
Bax, 37
Bcl-2, 37, 46, 81
Bcl-xL, 81
beneficial effect, 40
benign, 59
beta, 5, 80, 81
beta cell, 5, 81
biliary cirrhosis, 56
binding, 1, 5, 9, 11, 15, 21, 57, 65, 69, 70
bioactive, vii, 39
biological, 40, 97
biologically, 22
biology, 45, 67, 91
biopsies, 52, 62, 72, 96
biopsy, 32, 41, 57, 95
biosynthesis, 69
blocks, 36, 81
blood, 4, 38, 44, 68, 90
blood glucose, 44
blood pressure, 4, 90
blot, 72
body mass index (BMI), 1, 18, 32, 38
body weight, 41, 90
bone, 22
bone marrow, 22
bowel, 39, 82
brain, 67
breakdown, 6
buffer, 15
bypass, 38, 81, 82

C

caloric intake, 17, 28
calorie, 17, 82
cancer, 29, 33, 59, 94
candidates, 25
capacity, vii, 15, 21, 25, 31, 54
capillary, 74
carbohydrate, 1, 15, 33, 53, 68, 70, 79, 83
carbohydrate metabolism, 70
carbohydrates, 13, 17
carbon, 20, 31, 42
carbon dioxide, 20, 31
carbon tetrachloride, 42
carcinogens, 31, 33
carcinoma, viii, 1, 3, 26, 49, 61, 62, 93, 94
carcinomas, 81, 94
cardiovascular, 17
cardiovascular risk, 17
caspase, 45, 75
caspases, 37, 46
catabolism, 5, 6, 12, 16
catalase, 21, 56
catalysts, 73
cathepsin B, 37
Caucasians, 55
causal relationship, 30
cell, 4, 27, 34, 35, 43, 45, 50, 76, 77, 78, 80, 81, 86, 91, 92, 93, 96
cell cycle, 50
cell death, 45, 81
cell line, 78
cell surface, 4, 43
cellular immunity, 44
central obesity, 56
chemical, 77
children, 53, 77
cholesterol, 4, 67, 69
chromatin, 37
chromatography, 12
chromosome, 9
chronic, 3, 5, 18, 22, 50, 55, 59, 61, 76, 81, 82, 84, 92, 96
circulation, vii, 6, 7, 11, 12, 13, 14, 18, 22, 36, 39, 51

cirrhosis, viii, 3, 4, 23, 26, 27, 30, 35, 40, 45, 49, 50, 55, 56, 59, 62, 94, 96
clinical, 17, 21, 30, 39, 48, 62, 64, 79, 95, 96
clinical trial, 30
clinical trials, 30
clinicopathologic, 51
cloning, 84
clustering, 55
Co, 56
coding, 18
coenzyme, 95
cohort, 32, 34, 56
collagen, 2, 5, 9, 29, 33, 47, 48, 78, 84, 93
complement, 57
complementary, 5
complications, 3
components, 1, 5, 34, 44, 47, 57
composition, 17, 35, 70
concentration, 10, 12, 14, 31, 33, 34, 36, 45, 82, 88
condensation, 37
Congress, iv
conjugation, 76
connective tissue, 1, 48, 92
consensus, 40
consumption, viii, 3, 53
control, 23, 35, 37, 38, 40, 45, 62, 66, 68, 83
controlled, 72
conversion, 14
copper, 56
corn, 28, 29
coronary heart disease, 83
correlation, 22, 32, 33, 35, 36, 37, 41
correlations, 30
coupling, 21
CPTs, 36
C-reactive protein, 1, 7, 23, 74, 75
cross-sectional, 55
cross-sectional study, 55
cross-talk, 4
CRP, 1, 7
crystalline, 1, 30, 35, 79
crystals, 35
culture, 40, 48, 64, 70
Curcumin, 10, 67

Index

cysts, 53
cytochrome, viii, 1, 13, 21, 29, 32, 35, 37, 46, 72, 73, 74, 76, 78
cytokeratins, 54
cytokine, viii, 1, 10, 27, 30, 36, 40, 43, 44, 46, 48, 49, 86, 91
cytokines, 7, 8, 10, 11, 22, 26, 30, 39, 44, 47, 48, 53, 56, 59, 88, 91, 95
cytoplasm, 12, 52
cytosol, 37
cytosolic, 57
cytotoxic, viii, 30, 59

D

de novo, vii, 1, 11, 12, 13, 14, 38, 42, 59, 68
death, 45, 46, 81, 92
defects, 4, 9, 28, 36, 63, 81
defense, 57, 88
deficiency, 19, 28, 31, 34, 36, 41, 42, 44, 52, 67, 86, 91, 93, 94
degradation, 6, 11, 12, 18, 19, 32, 47, 67, 70
degree, 15, 21, 35, 42, 47, 48
dehydrogenase, 56, 78
delivery, 12, 13
delta, 1, 7, 65
demand, 3
density, 1, 13, 16, 68, 71
dephosphorylation, 5
deposition, 49
deposits, 53
detection, 77
detoxification, 57
developed nations, 4
diabetes, 8, 21, 31, 38, 40, 48, 49, 53, 55, 62, 63, 64, 66, 68, 69, 71, 72, 74, 78, 80, 81, 83, 85, 88, 89, 90, 91, 94, 95, 96, 97
diabetes mellitus, 55, 66, 68, 69, 80, 85, 89, 94, 96
diabetic, 10, 21, 27, 32, 34, 48, 53, 71, 72, 73, 77, 87, 95
diabetic patients, 10, 34, 87
diacylglycerol, 66
diagnostic, 49
diagnostic criteria, 49
diet, 8, 10, 11, 15, 17, 22, 27, 28, 29, 31, 32, 36, 44, 46, 47, 65, 66, 67, 68, 69, 73, 76, 86
dietary, 8, 12, 13, 14, 16, 17, 28, 33, 37, 45, 70, 76
dietary fat, 14, 16, 17
diets, 28, 68
differentiation, 5, 43, 44, 90
diseases, 27, 35, 52, 76
disorder, vii
displacement, 52
disposition, 13
dissociation, 31
distribution, 21, 37, 79, 96
DNA, 16, 30, 34, 35, 37, 50, 56, 77
DNA damage, 30, 35, 77
DNA repair, 50, 56
docosahexaenoic acid, 71
donors, 35
down-regulation, viii, 8, 57
drug targets, 80
drugs, 31, 52
duration, 41
dysfunctional, viii, 30, 31
dyslipidemia, 71
dysregulated, vii, 7, 22, 59
dysregulation, 15

E

ECM, 1, 47
efficacy, 77, 93
electron, 31, 35, 36
electron microscopy, 35
electronic, iv
electrons, 20, 21, 31
electrostatic, iv
emigration, 45
encoding, 22, 57
endocrine, 39
endogenous, 20, 31, 40
endoplasmic reticulum, 8, 16, 17, 18, 21, 29, 31
endothelium, 17
energy, 3, 20, 28, 36, 39, 40, 59, 63, 78, 83, 86

enlargement, 40
environmental, 15, 31, 48, 51, 54
environmental conditions, 15
environmental factors, 48, 51, 54
enzymatic, 19
enzyme, 20, 21, 28, 31, 34, 35, 37, 69
enzymes, 5, 6, 10, 16, 20, 21, 22, 29, 35, 41, 43, 45, 57, 73, 75, 76
eosinophils, 53
epidemiologic studies, 55
epidemiology, 64
equilibrium, 4
esterification, 20
esters, 17, 95
ethanol, 26, 38, 73, 78, 82
ethnic groups, 55
ethnicity, 55, 62
etiology, 53, 70
evidence, 3, 15, 23, 29, 30, 32, 33, 35, 42, 54, 55, 56, 63, 79, 84, 85
evolution, 48, 77
exogenous, 19, 41
exons, 69
expert, iv
exposure, 48, 52
extracellular, 1, 26, 30, 47, 84
extracellular matrix, 1, 47, 84
extrinsic, 46

F

factor-α∀, 74, 89
FAD, 20
failure, 4, 6, 62
familial, 55, 72
familial aggregation, 55
family, 16, 22, 31, 32, 37, 45, 88
Fas, 26, 45, 46, 92
fasting, 4, 12, 14, 16, 17, 20, 25, 32, 33, 41, 56, 72, 76
fasting glucose, 4, 32, 33, 41
fat, v, vii, 3, 6, 8, 10, 11, 12, 13, 14, 15, 16, 17, 22, 25, 26, 28, 29, 31, 32, 34, 36, 39, 41, 42, 45, 47, 52, 53, 59, 64, 66, 67, 68, 69, 70, 73, 74, 76, 83, 87, 93

fats, 15, 17, 18
fatty acid, vii, 1, 2, 5, 6, 7, 8, 9, 11, 12, 13, 14, 15, 16, 17, 18, 19, 20, 21, 22, 25, 26, 28, 31, 32, 34, 35, 36, 37, 38, 39, 41, 42, 43, 44, 46, 48, 50, 51, 56, 59, 63, 65, 66, 67, 68, 69, 70, 71, 74, 76, 79, 81
fatty acids, vii, 1, 2, 6, 7, 8, 9, 12, 13, 14, 15, 16, 17, 18, 19, 20, 21, 22, 31, 32, 34, 36, 38, 39, 42, 43, 48, 51, 59, 63, 66, 68, 71, 79, 81
fatty liver, 1, 3, 25, 35, 37, 38, 45, 50, 68, 71, 75, 85
feedback, 11
feeding, 15, 16, 19, 25, 28, 80
females, 56
ferritin, 33
fetal, 70
fibrate, 80
fibrinogen, 19, 57
fibroblasts, 93
fibrogenesis, v, 40, 45, 47, 48, 49, 57, 76, 84, 92
fibrosis, 4, 17, 23, 25, 26, 27, 28, 30, 34, 39, 40, 41, 42, 47, 48, 49, 51, 55, 59, 63, 68, 75, 77, 78, 79, 84, 85, 92, 93, 96
fish, 80
fish oil, 80
flora, 38, 82
flow, 36
food, 28, 40
food intake, 28, 40
fragmentation, 37
fructose, 14

G

gas, 12
gas chromatograph, 12
gender, 18, 50, 82
gene, 1, 5, 6, 10, 11, 16, 18, 19, 29, 32, 33, 40, 41, 48, 49, 56, 57, 72, 76, 78, 84, 85, 86, 87, 93, 97
gene expression, 5, 6, 10, 11, 16, 32, 48, 56, 87, 93, 97
generation, viii, 20, 26, 31

genes, 16, 22, 29, 35, 40, 47, 50, 56, 57, 69, 71, 97
genetic, 4, 10, 33, 34, 44, 48, 51, 52, 54, 55, 56, 80
genetic abnormalities, 34
genetic defect, 4
genetic factors, 48
genetic mutations, 33
genome, vii
genomic, 34, 97
gluconeogenesis, 6
glucose, 1, 4, 5, 6, 8, 11, 12, 14, 15, 16, 28, 29, 32, 33, 37, 39, 41, 42, 43, 44, 48, 56, 59, 63, 64, 66, 68, 69, 74, 81, 83, 87, 88, 91, 92
glucose metabolism, 37, 56, 66
glucose tolerance, 42, 44
GLUT, 1, 5
GLUT4, 5, 6, 8, 43, 63
glutathione, 36, 57
glycerol, 14
glycogen, 6, 51, 53, 65
glycogen synthase kinase, 65
glycolysis, 16, 70
glycoprotein, 45
goals, 63
grading, 54
groups, 38, 55, 56, 57
growth, 1, 5, 11, 37, 48, 57, 77, 88, 92, 93
growth factor, 1, 11, 48, 57, 77, 92, 93
gut, viii, 13, 16, 26, 38, 91

H

harmful, 12, 15, 17, 36, 54
harmful effects, 36
HDL, 4
health, 4
heart, 83, 97
heart disease, 83
heat, 1
heat shock protein, 1
hematopoiesis, 85
hemochromatosis, 1, 33
hepatic fibrosis, 27, 34, 42, 47, 59, 68, 84, 93
hepatic injury, 44
hepatic stellate cells, 1, 27, 40, 78, 84, 93
hepatitis, 35, 49, 55, 56, 84, 94, 95
hepatitis C, 35, 49, 55, 56, 84, 94
hepatocarcinogenesis, 74
hepatocellular, v, vii, viii, 1, 3, 15, 25, 26, 28, 36, 44, 49, 59, 61, 62, 81, 93, 94
hepatocellular carcinoma, viii, 1, 3, 26, 49, 61, 62, 81, 93, 94
hepatocyte, 17, 21, 22, 28, 29, 30, 31, 34, 36, 37, 39, 45, 46, 50, 52, 53, 54, 57, 73
hepatocytes, vii, 3, 4, 7, 12, 15, 18, 19, 21, 25, 26, 30, 31, 32, 35, 36, 37, 39, 45, 46, 50, 51, 52, 53, 54, 70, 78, 80, 90, 91
hepatoma, 19, 33, 50, 78
hepatomegaly, 42
high-fat, 8, 10, 11, 15, 22, 28, 29, 31, 32, 36, 45, 47, 67, 68, 73
Hispanics, 55
histological, 4, 28, 29, 30, 51, 62, 95
histology, 50
histopathology, 55, 97
homeostasis, 5, 63, 79, 83, 87
homolog, 9
homology, 1, 5, 9, 10
Honda, 84, 93
hormone, 6, 12, 13, 28, 40, 41, 76, 91
hormones, 31, 39, 83
HSC, 1, 27, 33, 40, 47, 48, 57
HSP, 1, 54
human, 1, 4, 5, 7, 10, 11, 16, 22, 27, 28, 29, 33, 41, 42, 43, 48, 49, 50, 66, 69, 71, 77, 78, 79, 81, 83, 84, 85, 86, 87, 88, 89, 90, 92, 93
human subjects, 11, 22, 41, 42, 43
humans, 5, 7, 14, 19, 21, 22, 27, 28, 31, 38, 41, 42, 43, 44, 54, 68, 77, 78, 81, 83, 86, 88, 91
hyaline, 51
hydrogen, 22, 31
hydrogen peroxide, 22, 31
hydroperoxides, 19
hydroxyl, 22, 31
hydroxylation, 77
hyperglycemia, 15, 33, 40, 48

Index

hyperinsulinemia, 3, 5, 6, 11, 14, 18, 25, 29, 36, 40, 42, 51, 88, 92
hyperlipidemia, 27
hypersensitivity, 28
hypertension, 4, 92
hypertensive, 49
hypertriglyceridemia, 11, 68
hypothalamus, 40, 41, 84
hypothesis, 30
hypoxemia, 32

I

id, 37, 40
IgG, 23
IL-1, 22, 27, 29, 40, 44, 48
IL-10, 27, 48
IL-15, 44
IL-6, 7, 10, 22, 29, 39, 44, 91
imaging, 56
immune cells, 44
immune response, 76, 85
immune system, 83, 91
immunity, 27, 44, 85
immunodeficiency, 85
immunohistochemistry, 72
immuno-regulatory, 91
immunosuppression, 76
in vitro, 18, 48, 88, 91
in vivo, 18, 32, 48, 74, 78, 88, 91
inactivation, 8, 11, 15, 29, 76
incidence, 49, 50
Indian, 88
Indians, 42
indicators, 54
indices, 30
indirect effect, 37
induction, 28, 41, 44, 45, 72, 75
infection, 43
inflammation, vii, 10, 12, 17, 22, 23, 26, 28, 29, 39, 41, 42, 43, 44, 45, 47, 49, 51, 53, 57, 59, 67, 73, 74, 75, 80, 83, 85, 87
inflammatory, 10, 23, 39, 41, 42, 45, 46, 50, 53, 66, 82, 86
inflammatory mediators, 10

inflammatory response, 42
infusions, 10, 43
inheritance, 55
inhibition, 5, 10, 11, 28, 37, 41, 42, 43, 54, 65, 95
inhibitor, 1, 7, 9, 10, 46
inhibitory, 6, 7
inhibitory effect, 6
injury, iv, v, viii, 17, 21, 25, 26, 28, 29, 30, 34, 35, 36, 37, 40, 44, 46, 48, 50, 52, 59, 69, 70, 75, 81, 82, 84, 92, 96
iNOS, 1, 10, 11, 22
inositol, 1, 5, 9
insulin, vii, 1, 2, 3, 4, 5, 6, 7, 8, 9, 10, 11, 12, 14, 15, 16, 18, 20, 21, 22, 23, 25, 26, 27, 28, 29, 31, 32, 34, 36, 38, 39, 40, 41, 42, 43, 44, 48, 49, 51, 54, 56, 59, 62, 63, 64, 65, 66, 67, 68, 69, 71, 72, 74, 75, 76, 79, 80, 81, 82, 83, 85, 87, 88, 89, 90, 91, 97
insulin resistance, vii, 2, 3, 5, 7, 8, 9, 10, 11, 12, 14, 15, 20, 22, 25, 26, 27, 28, 29, 32, 33, 34, 36, 38, 39, 40, 41, 42, 43, 44, 48, 49, 51, 54, 56, 59, 62, 63, 64, 65, 66, 67, 69, 71, 74, 75, 76, 79, 80, 83, 85, 87, 88, 89, 90, 91, 97
insulin sensitivity, 7, 10, 11, 23, 34, 39, 40, 42, 44, 50, 57, 90
insulin signaling, vii, 4, 5, 6, 7, 9, 10, 40, 42, 59, 65, 67
insulin-like growth factor, 57
insults, 27
integrity, 39
interaction, 39, 68, 93, 96
interactions, 38, 82
interference, 5
interleukin, 1, 7, 90, 91
interleukin-6, 7, 90, 91
interpretation, 95
interval, 41
intracellular signaling, 36, 41
intravenous, 10
intrinsic, 4, 37
iron, 19, 26, 30, 33, 47, 49, 51, 63, 78, 79
iron deficiency, 34
IRS, 1, 5, 7, 8, 9, 10, 11, 15, 64, 65

isoforms, 10, 21, 28, 31
isotope, 12, 14, 71
isotopes, 71
Italy, 61

J

Japan, 61
JNK, 1, 7, 8, 9, 10, 15, 65
Jun, 1, 7, 9

K

kappa, 1, 10
kappa B, 1, 10
kinase, 1, 4, 7, 9, 11, 16, 40, 41, 42, 64, 65, 66, 88, 89
kinase activity, 4, 65
kinases, 8, 9
knockout, 8, 11, 27, 42

L

L1, 87
lambda, 65
L-carnitine, 80
LDL, 13
lead, 19, 26, 59
leptin, 1, 8, 11, 27, 29, 38, 39, 40, 41, 42, 44, 48, 56, 67, 75, 76, 80, 83, 84, 85, 86, 89, 91
lesions, 30
leukocytes, 53
lice, 64
ligand, 26, 43, 45, 90
ligands, 46
limitation, 14
links, vii, 67, 80, 91
linoleic acid, 70
lipase, 5, 12, 13, 43, 89
lipases, 16, 17
lipid, vii, viii, 5, 6, 9, 11, 19, 20, 23, 25, 28, 29, 30, 34, 35, 38, 39, 46, 47, 48, 52, 53, 54, 56, 59, 65, 68, 70, 71, 72, 73, 75, 77, 80, 81, 83, 87, 88, 92, 93

lipid metabolism, 5, 6, 39, 83, 88
lipid peroxidation, vii, viii, 19, 23, 25, 28, 29, 30, 34, 35, 47, 53, 59, 73, 75, 77, 93
lipid peroxides, 28, 73
lipids, vii, 5, 13, 20, 39, 71
lipodystrophy, 40, 41, 55, 69, 83, 85, 86, 96
lipolysis, vii, 5, 6, 12, 14, 22, 31, 43, 59, 64
lipophilic, 31
lipopolysaccharide, 1, 26, 27, 81
lipoprotein, 2, 5, 12, 16, 17, 22, 43, 68, 71, 89
lipoproteins, vii, 1, 13, 16, 68, 70
liposuction, 40, 83
literature, vii, 15
liver, v, vii, viii, 1, 3, 4, 5, 6, 8, 11, 12, 13, 14, 15, 16, 17, 18, 19, 20, 21, 22, 25, 27, 28, 29, 32, 33, 35, 36, 37, 38, 39, 40, 41, 42, 44, 45, 47, 48, 49, 52, 55, 59, 61, 62, 63, 64, 66, 67, 68, 69, 70, 71, 72, 73, 74, 75, 76, 77, 79, 80, 81, 82, 84, 85, 89, 91, 92, 93, 94, 95, 96, 97
liver cancer, 29, 33, 59
liver cells, 16
liver damage, 82, 91
liver disease, vii, 1, 3, 4, 33, 35, 38, 55, 59, 61, 62, 63, 66, 68, 69, 70, 72, 73, 74, 75, 76, 77, 79, 82, 84, 85, 89, 91, 92, 94, 95, 96, 97
liver enzymes, 45, 75
liver failure, 4, 62
liver transplant, 38
liver transplantation, 38
localization, 32
location, 39, 47
London, 61
longitudinal study, 62, 96
low fat diet, 17
low-density, vii, 2, 6, 13, 17, 71
low-density lipoprotein, vii, 2, 6, 13, 17, 71
LPS, 1, 27, 38
lumen, 18, 82
lymphocyte, 32, 91
lymphocytes, 53, 72
lysosomes, 18, 37

M

macromolecules, 35
macronutrients, 5
macrophage, 22, 67, 95
macrophages, 7, 22, 39, 42, 53, 85, 88
magnetic, iv, 56
magnetic resonance, 56
magnetic resonance imaging, 56
malignancy, 43
malnutrition, 82, 85
malondialdehyde, 25, 30
management, 92, 97
manipulation, vii
manners, 43
MAPK, 1, 5
mapping, 86
marrow, 22
mass spectrometry, 12, 71
matrix, 1, 34, 35, 47, 84
maturation, 40
Maya, 78
MCP, 22
MCP-1, 22
meals, 20
measurement, 28, 70
mechanical, iv
mediators, 8, 9, 10, 27, 39, 45, 56, 57, 69
membranes, 30, 35, 36
men, 4, 63, 75, 90
messenger ribonucleic acid, 72
metabolic, 4, 6, 8, 18, 22, 25, 33, 37, 39, 40, 48, 54, 63, 64, 67, 69, 70, 72, 74, 75, 76, 80, 83, 86, 87, 97
metabolic dysfunction, 86
metabolic pathways, 37
metabolic syndrome, 4, 25, 54, 63, 64, 67, 69, 74, 75, 80, 83, 86, 87, 97
metabolism, 5, 6, 21, 22, 37, 39, 56, 64, 65, 66, 69, 70, 71, 78, 81, 83, 88
metabolites, 9, 15
methionine, 1, 10, 27, 76
mice, 5, 7, 8, 10, 11, 14, 16, 19, 22, 25, 27, 28, 29, 32, 36, 37, 38, 40, 42, 43, 44, 48, 50, 67, 68, 69, 73, 74, 75, 76, 77, 80, 84, 85, 87, 89, 91, 92, 93, 94, 95
microcirculation, 92
microscopy, 35
minority, viii
MIP, 29
misfolded, 54, 96
mitochondria, viii, 20, 29, 30, 31, 34, 35, 36, 37, 41, 46, 66, 72, 81
mitochondrial, 1, 2, 6, 8, 13, 16, 20, 21, 22, 26, 28, 30, 31, 32, 34, 35, 36, 37, 41, 42, 46, 51, 52, 56, 59, 63, 72, 79, 80, 81, 92, 95
mitochondrial abnormalities, 34, 35, 63
mitochondrial damage, 37
mitochondrial DNA, 34, 35, 57
mitochondrial membrane, 16, 30, 81
mitogen, 1, 5
mitogen-activated protein kinase, 1, 5
models, vii, 8, 19, 21, 22, 27, 28, 29, 39, 43, 44, 47, 49, 76
moieties, 20
molecular oxygen, 22, 31
molecules, 9, 16, 20, 22, 64
monocyte, 7, 88
monocytes, 41, 85
mononuclear cell, 45
mononuclear cells, 45
monounsaturated fat, 14
Monroe, 84
morphological, 51
motion, 26
mouse, vii, 27, 46, 66, 67, 69, 76, 84, 85, 86
mRNA, 11, 21, 29, 32, 42, 43, 47, 48, 80
multi-ethnic, 55
murine model, 28, 37
muscle, vii, 1, 4, 6, 7, 8, 11, 15, 22, 32, 34, 40, 42, 43, 47, 66, 67, 74, 87
muscle cells, 34, 40, 42
muscle relaxant, 32
muscles, 7, 8, 11, 35
musculoskeletal, 87
mutagenesis, 64
mutant, 29
mutation, 40, 41, 50, 57, 86
mutations, 18, 19, 33, 63, 72, 78, 79

N

NAD, 20
NADH, 20, 21
natural, viii, 1, 27, 40, 61, 62, 79, 93, 96
natural killer, viii, 1, 27
necrosis, 2, 7, 9, 45, 54, 65, 66, 67, 74, 75, 81, 82, 87, 89, 90, 92, 97
neoplasia, 29, 76
nervous system, 40
network, 26, 34
neural network, 85, 86
neural networks, 85, 86
neuroendocrine, 86
neuropeptide, 41
neurotransmitter, 27
New York, iii, iv
NF-κB, 1, 10, 37, 46
nitric oxide, 1, 10, 11, 67, 68, 74
nitric oxide synthase, 1, 10, 67, 68, 74
non-alcoholic fatty liver, 66, 68, 69, 75, 77, 84
nonalcoholic steatohepatitis (NASH), viii, 3
non-enzymatic, 19
noradrenaline, 45
norepinephrine, 49
normal, 18, 19, 21, 31, 33, 35, 36, 42, 44, 45, 54, 63, 83
normal conditions, 31, 54
normalization, 11
N-terminal, 1, 7, 9
nuclear, 1, 10, 22, 34, 69
nuclei, 51, 53, 95
nucleus, 10, 16, 52
nutrition, 80, 82

O

obese, 7, 8, 10, 12, 13, 14, 15, 18, 20, 21, 22, 25, 27, 28, 32, 34, 36, 38, 41, 45, 48, 50, 53, 55, 57, 67, 68, 70, 72, 73, 75, 77, 80, 83, 84, 85, 87, 89, 90, 97
obese patients, 7, 12, 15, 20, 32, 53, 55, 57, 77, 89, 97
obesity, vii, 4, 8, 10, 17, 21, 22, 27, 28, 29, 31, 36, 38, 40, 42, 43, 44, 48, 49, 51, 55, 62, 63, 65, 66, 67, 68, 69, 74, 75, 80, 83, 84, 86, 88, 89, 90, 91, 95, 97
observations, 27, 32, 34, 36, 38, 57
oil, 28, 29, 80
oils, 71
olive, 28
oral, 32
organ, 11, 23, 37, 72, 74
organelles, 34
overload, 8, 21, 30, 51
overproduction, 71
overweight, 48, 92
oxidation, vii, 6, 12, 13, 16, 20, 21, 22, 26, 28, 31, 32, 34, 35, 36, 41, 42, 50, 59, 72, 74, 76, 87, 88
oxidative, vii, viii, 2, 8, 19, 22, 23, 25, 27, 29, 30, 33, 34, 35, 38, 41, 50, 51, 53, 57, 59, 73, 74, 77, 78
oxidative damage, 19
oxidative stress, vii, viii, 2, 8, 19, 22, 23, 25, 27, 29, 30, 33, 34, 35, 38, 41, 50, 51, 53, 57, 59, 73, 74, 77, 78
oxide, 1, 10, 11, 67, 68, 74
oxygen, 20, 21, 22, 31, 73

P

Pacific, 77
pancreas, 11
pancreatic, 6, 81
paracrine, 7, 43, 47
paraffin-embedded, 32
parenteral, 80, 82
particles, 17
pathogenesis, v, vii, viii, 19, 25, 27, 30, 31, 33, 39, 43, 48, 50, 51, 56, 57, 75, 76, 77, 80, 82, 85, 89, 95, 96
pathogenic, 68
pathology, 52, 59, 95
pathophysiological, vii, 34, 83
pathophysiology, 4, 27, 29, 54, 57, 92

pathways, 5, 13, 18, 19, 21, 36, 41, 50, 54, 71, 81, 82
patients, viii, 3, 7, 8, 10, 11, 12, 14, 15, 16, 17, 18, 19, 20, 21, 23, 26, 30, 32, 33, 34, 35, 36, 38, 39, 41, 42, 43, 45, 46, 47, 48, 49, 50, 52, 53, 54, 55, 56, 57, 62, 68, 69, 73, 75, 77, 79, 80, 86, 87, 89, 90, 92, 93, 94, 97
pediatric, 95
permeability, 36, 38, 82
peroxidation, vii, viii, 14, 19, 23, 25, 28, 29, 30, 34, 35, 47, 48, 53, 59, 70, 71, 73, 75, 77, 92, 93
peroxide, 22, 31
Peroxisome, 22, 74
peroxisomes, 16, 21, 26, 30, 31
phagocytic, 39, 42
phenotype, 95
phenotypic, 27
Philadelphia, 74
phlebotomies, 34
phosphatases, 8, 9
phosphate, 14
phospholipids, 17
phosphorylates, 8, 9, 10, 40
phosphorylation, 5, 7, 8, 9, 10, 11, 15, 34, 35, 40, 64, 65, 89, 95
physiological, 5, 7, 54
PI3K, 50
pilot study, 38, 77, 79, 90
pioglitazone, 87, 90
pituitary, 86
plasma, vii, 5, 6, 7, 9, 12, 13, 14, 15, 16, 17, 18, 19, 33, 38, 40, 41, 42, 43, 44, 48, 49, 59, 68, 71, 80, 83, 85, 86, 87, 88, 89
plasma levels, 40, 42
plasma membrane, 5
platelet, 35
play, 5, 7, 10, 29, 30, 31, 32, 33, 39, 57, 84
polarization, viii, 44
polygenic, 96
polymorphism, 97
polymorphisms, 57, 97
polymorphonuclear, 53
polypeptide, 40, 41

polyunsaturated fat, 1, 17, 18, 69
polyunsaturated fatty acid, 1, 17, 18, 69
polyunsaturated fatty acids, 1, 17, 18
poor, 7
population, 23, 33, 55, 61, 62, 88
portal hypertension, 92
positive correlation, 22, 32, 37, 41
positive relation, 9, 45
positive relationship, 9, 45
postmenopausal, 83
postmenopausal women, 83
predictors, 32, 54
pregnancy, 52
preparation, iv
pressure, 4, 90
prevention, 81, 82
preventive, 3, 27
primary biliary cirrhosis, 56
probe, 32
probiotics, 39, 82
producers, 21
production, vii, viii, 5, 7, 10, 11, 15, 21, 22, 27, 30, 31, 33, 34, 35, 36, 38, 42, 43, 44, 48, 50, 51, 54, 56, 59, 63, 64, 68, 70, 71, 82, 84, 88, 91
progenitors, 88
prognostic factors, 68
program, 67
progressive, 4, 33, 52, 59, 96, 97
proinflammatory, viii, 7, 8, 9, 10, 11, 30, 39, 41, 43, 44, 47, 48, 53, 56, 59, 85
proliferation, 22, 28, 29, 43, 85
promote, 6, 8, 22, 30, 34, 36, 38, 46, 53, 80
promoter, 18, 57, 97
property, iv
protection, 15, 56
protective mechanisms, 20
protein, 1, 5, 7, 9, 10, 11, 16, 18, 21, 23, 32, 35, 36, 37, 41, 42, 43, 48, 54, 57, 65, 69, 70, 71, 74, 75, 79, 80, 81, 82, 85, 86, 88, 97
protein kinase C, 1, 7, 65
protein synthesis, 41
proteins, 5, 9, 10, 34, 37, 39, 40, 54, 57, 67, 69, 81, 96
proteolysis, 1, 18, 69

PUFA, 19
PUFAs, 1, 18, 19, 30
pyruvate, 16

R

race, 56
radical, 22, 31
rat, 19, 28, 32, 33, 37, 70, 72, 73, 74, 78, 82, 84, 92, 93
rats, 8, 11, 15, 17, 19, 27, 28, 32, 33, 47, 48, 64, 67, 71, 72, 73, 77, 80, 93
reactive oxygen, viii, 1, 10, 20, 21, 31
reactive oxygen species (ROS), viii, 2, 10, 20, 31
receptors, 39, 41, 43, 44, 65, 74, 75, 87, 89, 92
reduction, 16, 20, 73, 78
reflection, 45
regenerative capacity, 25
regulation, viii, 5, 8, 10, 11, 12, 17, 32, 36, 44, 56, 57, 63, 64, 69, 71, 77, 78, 80, 82, 83, 85, 87, 90, 96
relationship, 9, 15, 30, 33, 35, 38, 42, 45, 47, 48, 68, 86, 89, 95
relationships, 80
remodeling, 84
renin, 49
renin-angiotensin system, 49
repair, 50, 57
repair system, 50
research, viii, 17, 67
researchers, 22
residues, 7, 8, 9
resistance, vii, 2, 3, 4, 5, 6, 7, 8, 9, 10, 11, 12, 13, 14, 15, 16, 18, 20, 22, 25, 26, 27, 28, 29, 32, 33, 34, 36, 37, 39, 40, 41, 42, 43, 44, 48, 49, 51, 55, 56, 59, 62, 63, 64, 65, 66, 67, 69, 71, 74, 75, 76, 79, 80, 83, 85, 87, 88, 89, 90, 91, 97
resistin, 39, 44, 91
respiration, 31
respiratory, 1, 20, 79
retention, 18, 19
reticulum, 1, 8, 16, 17, 18, 21, 29, 31
ribonucleic acid, 72

risk, 3, 42, 49, 55, 62, 74, 83
risk factors, 3, 55, 62, 75, 83
risks, 17, 55
RNA, 29
rodent, 19
rodents, 8, 41, 43
ROS, 1, 10, 15, 16, 20, 21, 22, 30, 31, 34, 35, 36, 39, 45, 48, 57
rosiglitazone, 90

S

salicylates, 10, 23, 65
sample, 55
sarcoidosis, 55
saturated fat, 15, 17, 18, 37, 66
saturated fatty acids, 17, 18, 66
saturation, 33
scavenger, 88
scores, 41
secrete, 22, 47
secretion, vii, 12, 16, 17, 18, 19, 41, 44, 46, 70, 71, 81, 87, 91
sensitivity, viii, 7, 10, 11, 23, 34, 39, 40, 42, 44, 50, 57, 67, 75, 90
sensitization, 82, 91
sequelae, 87
serine, 2, 7, 8, 9, 64, 65
serum, 17, 27, 28, 29, 33, 38, 41, 42, 45, 61, 63, 79, 84, 88, 89, 90
serum transferrin, 33
services, iv
severity, 17, 25, 32, 35, 47, 48, 62, 67, 76, 79
sex, 18, 23, 28, 32, 38
shock, 1
signal transduction, 2, 9, 11, 44, 66
signal(l)ing, vii, 2, 4, 5, 6, 7, 8, 9, 10, 36, 38, 39, 40, 41, 42, 59, 64, 65, 67, 78, 81, 84, 87, 91
signaling pathway, 5, 36, 41, 81
signaling pathways, 5, 36, 41, 81
signals, 27
similarity, 14, 18, 28, 54
sites, 5, 31, 40
skeletal muscle, vii, 4, 6, 8, 32, 34, 43, 66, 74

SMA, 47
smooth muscle, 1, 47
SOD, 57
species, viii, 2, 10, 20, 22, 31
spectrum, 59, 62, 97
Sprague-Dawley rats, 28
stages, 35, 49, 54, 57
starvation, 4, 76
steatosis, vii, 4, 11, 15, 18, 23, 27, 28, 29, 30, 32, 35, 36, 41, 42, 43, 45, 47, 51, 52, 54, 55, 57, 59, 62, 65, 67, 69, 71, 73, 75, 76, 77, 79, 82, 90, 92, 95, 97
stellate cells, 1, 27, 40, 47, 78, 84, 92, 93
steroid, 31
steroid hormone, 31
steroid hormones, 31
stimulus, 17
stoichiometry, 73
storage, 5, 15, 36, 39
strain, 27
strategies, 3, 27
stress, vii, viii, 2, 8, 10, 13, 19, 20, 21, 22, 23, 25, 28, 29, 30, 31, 32, 33, 34, 35, 38, 41, 45, 48, 50, 51, 53, 54, 57, 59, 66, 70, 73, 74, 75, 77, 78, 96
stressors, 54
subacute, 4, 10
substances, 2, 19
substrates, vii, 5, 7, 9, 11, 21, 31, 64
sucrose, 28, 45
sugar, 33, 78
sugars, 17
Sun, 70
superoxide, 22, 31, 56
superoxide dismutase, 56
supply, 15, 25
suppression, 11, 63, 65, 68
suppressors, 2, 10, 67
suppressors of cytokine signaling, 2, 10, 67
Surgery, 94, 97
surgical, 38, 39, 40
susceptibility, 36, 54, 56
swelling, 34
sympathetic, 40
sympathetic nervous system, 40

syndrome, 4, 25, 52, 54, 63, 64, 67, 69, 74, 75, 80, 83, 86, 87, 97
synthesis, vii, 5, 6, 11, 12, 14, 15, 16, 17, 18, 19, 20, 25, 31, 36, 41, 42, 43, 57, 59, 67, 68, 70, 71
systems, 21, 37, 50, 54, 56

T

T cell, viii, 1, 27, 45, 76, 86
T cells, viii, 1, 45
targets, 6, 10, 30, 80
tetracycline, 52
TGF, 1, 26, 40, 48, 49
therapeutic, 86
therapy, 41, 80, 85
theta, 1, 8
thiazolidinediones, 64
thiobarbituric acid, 2, 19
Thomson, 82
threat, 4, 71
threonine, 8, 65
thymus, 45
time, 15, 35, 37, 50, 52, 54, 59
TIMP, 47
TIMP-1, 47
tissue, vii, 1, 4, 5, 6, 7, 8, 12, 13, 14, 15, 18, 20, 22, 25, 39, 40, 41, 42, 43, 44, 48, 54, 67, 68, 69, 71, 80, 83, 85, 86, 87, 88, 89, 90, 91, 92
TNF, 2, 7, 8, 9, 10, 22, 26, 27, 28, 29, 30, 34, 36, 37, 38, 39, 40, 41, 42, 43, 45, 46, 49, 57, 65, 74, 75, 76, 80, 81, 82, 90
TNF-α, 2, 7, 8, 9, 10, 22, 26, 27, 28, 29, 30, 34, 36, 37, 38, 39, 40, 41, 42, 43, 45, 46, 49
tolerance, 42, 44
total parenteral nutrition, 82
toxic, 25
toxic products, 25
toxicity, 36, 37, 46, 51, 77
toxin, 52
toxins, 26, 31, 38, 52
transcription, 2, 10, 11, 16, 22, 29, 32, 40, 69, 70
transcription factor, 10, 16, 22, 69, 70

Index

transcription factors, 16, 22, 69
transcriptional, 37, 78
transduction, 2, 9, 11, 44, 66
transfer, 1, 18, 20, 36, 71, 97
transferrin, 33
transformation, 50
transforming growth factor, 2, 26, 77
transforming growth factor-β, 2, 26
transgenic, 69
transgenic mice, 69
translocation, 5, 10, 37
transmembrane, 40, 43, 44
transplantation, 38, 72
transport, 5, 6, 8, 17, 22, 31
tricarboxylic acid, 20
tricarboxylic acid cycle, 20
triglyceride, 1, 4, 5, 6, 12, 13, 14, 15, 16, 17, 18, 19, 20, 25, 28, 30, 42, 59, 68, 71, 97
triglycerides, vii, 3, 4, 7, 12, 14, 15, 16, 17, 18, 19, 20, 28, 41, 52, 59
tumo(u)r, 2, 7, 9, 49, 67, 74, 75, 82, 87, 89, 90, 92
tumor necrosis factor, 2, 7, 9, 67, 74, 75, 89, 90, 92
turnover, 45, 81
type 2 (II) diabetes, 4, 15, 21, 36, 42, 55, 64, 66, 80, 88, 89, 96, 97
type 2 diabetes mellitus, 4, 15, 21, 36, 42, 55
tyrosine, 4, 7, 8, 9, 11, 15, 65

U

ubiquitin, 54, 67
United States, 61, 62, 79, 94
urban, 62
urban population, 62

V

vacuole, 53
validation, 95

valproic acid, 52
variability, 35
variable, 4, 28, 55
variation, 77
vascular, 17
very low density lipoprotein, 68, 71
viral, 49
viral hepatitis, 49
vitamin C, 77
vitamin E, 19, 30
VLDL, 2, 6, 12, 13, 14, 16, 17, 18, 19, 20, 68, 70
vulnerability, 75

W

Washington, 92
water, 20, 31
Watson, 76
weight loss, 17, 22, 32, 40, 44, 70, 73, 87, 89, 90
Wilson's disease, 53
women, 4, 80, 83, 87, 90, 97

X
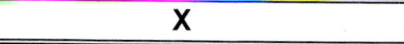

xenobiotic, 78
xenobiotics, 31

Y

young adults, 84

Z

Zen, 93
zinc, 56